The Case of the Unwanted Pounds

A Weight-Loss & Fitness Mystery

Fred A. Stutman, M.D.

MEDICAL MANOR BOOKS
PHILADELPHIA, PA

Medical Manor Books are available at special quantity discounts for sales promotions, premiums, fund raising or educational use. Book excerpts can also be created to fit special needs.

For details write the
Special Markets Dept. of Medical Manor Books
3501 Newberry Road, Philadelphia, PA 19154

Phone: 800-DIETING (343-8464)
E-mail: info@medicalmanorbooks.com
Website: www.medicalmanorbooks.com

Other Books By The Author:

Walk, Don't Run. Philadelphia: Medical Manor Press, 1979.

The Doctor's Walking Book. New York: Ballantine Books, 1980.

The Doctor's Walking Diet. Philadelphia: Medical Manor Books, 1982.

DietWalk: The Doctor's Fast 3-Day SuperDiet. Philadelphia: Medical Manor Books, 1983. Pocket Books® Edition, Simon & Schuster, New York, 1987.

Walk, Don't Die. Philadelphia: Medical Manor Books, 1986. Bart Books Edition: New York, 1988.

Walk To Win: The Easy 4-Day Diet & Fitness Plan. Philadelphia: Medical Manor Books, 1990.

Diet-Step: 20/20-For Women Only. Philadelphia: Medical Manor Books, 2001.

Diet-Step: For Seniors. Philadelphia: Medical Manor Books, 2003.

100 Best Weight-Loss Tips. Philadelphia: Medical Manor Books, 2005.

100 Weight-Loss Tips That Really Work. New York: McGraw Hill Books, 2007.

Dr. Walk's Power Diet-Step. Philadelphia: Medical Manor Books, 2009.

Copyright© 2011 by Fred A. Stutman, M.D.

All Rights Reserved. No part of this book may be reproduced, copied or utilized in any form or by any means, electronic, mechanical, photocopying, recording, or by any information storage and retrieval system, without permission in writing from the publisher. Inquiries should be addressed to: Medical Manor Books, 3501 Newberry Road, Philadelphia, PA 19154.

Publisher's Cataloging-in-Publication
(Provided by Quality Books, Inc.)

Stutman, Fred A.
The case of the unwanted pounds : a weight-loss & fitness mystery / by Fred A. Stutman. -- 1st ed.
p. cm.
Includes index.
LCCN 2010916513
ISBN-13: 978-0-934232-26-5
ISBN-10: 0-934232-26-1

   1. Reducing diets. 2. Fitness walking.
  3. Nutrition. 4. Reducing exercises. I. Title.

RA222.2.S78 2011   613.2'5
              QBI10-600232

First Edition 2011

Manufactured in the United States of America

To:

Suzanne

Robert, Mary, Samantha, Alana

Roni, Paul, Geoffrey, Eddie

Craig, Christine, Rain, India

& Sparkey

Acknowledgements

EDITOR: Suzanne Stutman, Ph.D.

EDITORIAL STAFF: Patricia McGarvey, Mary Ann Johnston, Linda Quinn, Sheryl Bartkus, Patti Hartigan

PERMISSIONS: The American Academy of Family Practice; J & J Snack Foods, Inc.; The Physicians' Health Bulletin; Dr. Walk's Diet & Fitness Newsletter

WORD PROCESSING: Accu-Med Transcription Service

ILLUSTRATIONS: Steve Oswald, Norm Rockwell, Judit Meszaros

COVER DESIGN: Alexander E. Shin

TEXT DESIGN: Erin Howarth

PUBLISHER: Medical Manor Books, Philadelphia, PA

DR. WALK® is the registered trademark of Dr. Stutman's Diet & Fitness Newsletter. REG. U.S. PAT. OFF.

DIET-STEP® is the registered trademark of Dr. Stutman's Weight-Loss Program. REG. U.S. PAT. OFF.

FIT-STEP® is the registered trademark of Dr. Stutman's Fitness Walking Program. REG. U.S. PAT. OFF.

TRIM-STEP® is the registered trademark of Dr. Stutman's Stretching and Strength Training Program. REG. U.S. PAT. OFF.

POWER DIETSTEP® is the registered trademark of Dr. Stutman's Weight-Loss, Fitness & Body-Shaping Plan. REG. U.S. PAT. OFF.

Table of Contents

INTRODUCTION — ix

1. The Diet Fit-Step Mystery — 1
2. 21-Day Quick Weight-Loss Plan — 21
3. Fearless Fiber: Secret Agent — 49
4. Mr. Fat: Guilty of Murder! — 79
5. Dr. Walk's Mystery Diet Clues — 103
6. Get Fit & Trim in 35 Minutes — 135
7. Detective Walker Stays Slim — 161
8. Walk, Don't Die! — 187
9. Secret of Everlasting Youth — 215
10. Body-Shaping Mystery Solved — 235

APPENDIX
   Fat & Fiber Counter — 265

SUBJECT INDEX — 307

AUTHOR'S CAUTION

IT IS ESSENTIAL THAT YOU CONSULT YOUR OWN PHYSICIAN BEFORE BEGINNING THIS DIET AND FITNESS PLAN.

-Fred A. Stutman, M.D.

Introduction

*T**he Case of the Unwanted Pounds* presents a new, quick weight-loss formula, and an easy fitness and body-shaping plan, called *The Diet Fit-Step Mystery*. This unique program presents a series of clues that will show you how to lose weight, get fit, and re-shape your body quickly and safely. Your body will become thinner, your muscles and bones stronger and your figure firmer and shapelier. This quick weight-loss formula and easy body-shaping plan is formulated exclusively for those individuals who are tired of unhealthy, low-carbohydrate fad diets, and dangerous strenuous exercises.

This Diet Fit-Step Plan actually boosts your energy level and burns fat, while keeping you trim and fit. By combining a healthy easy-to-follow diet plan with an aerobic walking program and easy strength-training exercises, you will lose weight, become fit and build muscle quickly. This unique mystery combination delivers a double-blast of calorie burning for complete cardiovascular fitness, maximum weight-loss and complete body-shaping. And, believe it or not, you can actually lose up to 15 pounds and 3 inches in only 21 days.

The Diet Fit-Step Mystery was designed with you in mind. I originally formulated this weight-loss and fitness plan for my patients, who like most of you, really wanted a healthy and effective way to lose weight and get fit quickly. By utilizing these diet and fitness clues, you will be able to boost your energy level, lose weight, and build muscle in only 21 days. The weight you lose will stay lost forever and the fitness you gain will last you a lifetime. At last, a diet and exercise plan that really works and keeps on working. The Diet Fit-Step Mystery will show you how to slim down, shape-up, look younger and live longer. *You will finally be able to lose those unwanted pounds permanently.*

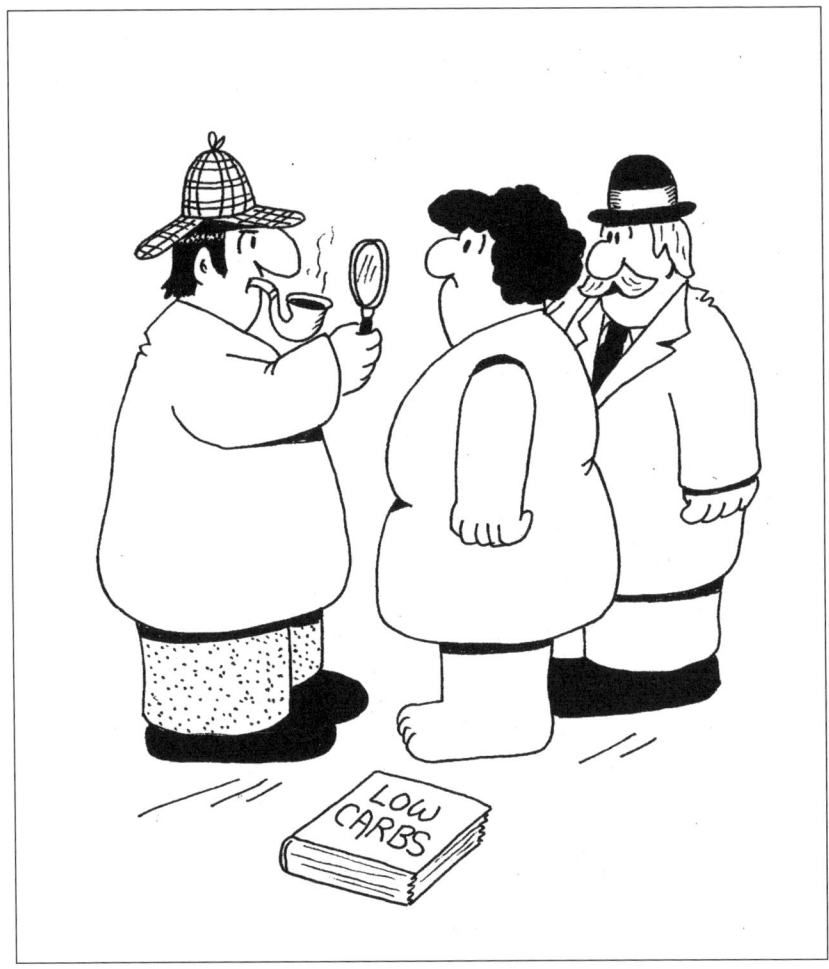

"My Dear Watson, how many times have I told these Americans to stay away from low carbohydrate diets?"

1

The Diet Fit-Step® Mystery

In *The Case of the Unwanted Pounds: A Weight-Loss & Fitness Mystery,* we present a series of clues in this unique diet and fitness mystery book. The mystery program presented in this book was designed for those individuals who are always on some sort of fad diet, and when they are through dieting, they always seem to still have unwanted pounds that actually never come off, no matter how hard they try to diet. Even more frustrating is the fact that once they have finished with the diet, they usually gain back more weight than they lost before they started the diet. This is called "rebound weight-gain," which is all too common with fad diets. Many people also think that strenuous exercises will help them lose weight and become fit, only to find that these types of exercises will not cause permanent weight loss or lasting fitness, and may in fact do more harm than good.

The clues presented in *The Case of the Unwanted Pounds* solve the mystery of how to lose weight quickly, and permanently, and how to achieve maximum cardiovascular fitness. These mystery clues also show you how to strengthen your muscles and bones, while shaping your body. In addition, this plan also helps you to live longer by preventing the degenerative diseases of aging, including heart attacks, hypertension, strokes and certain forms of cancer. The diet and fitness plan presented herein is called the *Diet Fit-Step Mystery*. This unique mystery program reveals the hazards of unhealthy fad diets and strenuous exercises, and illuminates the benefits of a truly healthy permanent weight-loss diet plan, and a safe and effective fitness plan. The Diet Fit-Step Plan shows you how to slim down, shape up, and look younger in just 21 days, and finally lose those unwanted pounds.

SHERLOCK HOLMES AND THE CASE OF THE NEFARIOUS DIET CHARLATANS

In the late 19th century London, it took the famous detective Sherlock Holmes to unmask a den of nefarious diet-scam charlatans and thieves from the very depths of London's seamier side. The notorious and devious organizer of these diet scams was a certain Professor James Moriarity, known in fact as "The Napoleon of Crime." His minions were found to be perpetrating a variation of the low carbohydrate diet scam on the unsuspecting, obese upper class inhabitants in London's posh neighborhoods. Moriarity created a spider's web of diet-scam charlatans throughout all of London. These scoundrels fleeced the well-to-do Londoners out of their money by selling them a bill-of-goods on the so-called weight-loss benefits of these dangerous low carbohydrate diets. These obese individuals were only too happy to consume mass quantities of beef, mutton, game, and cheese along with their beer and wine, while limiting their intake of healthy fresh vegetables and fruits.

It took the deductive and reasoning powers of Sherlock Holmes and the medical knowledge of Dr. Watson, to be able to convince these unfortunate, rotund individuals that they were putting their health and in fact, their very lives at considerable risk. Both Holmes and Watson informed these individuals that the weight that they initially lost was only water weight, and they were also told that any weight that they did lose initially would come back tenfold once they stopped the diet, provided they didn't die first.

Many a wealthy Londoner went to an early grave before Holmes was able to put a stop to this wicked scheme. As Sherlock Holmes once said to Dr. Watson, "It is an old maxim of mine that when you have excluded the impossible, whatever remains, however improbable, must be the truth." In a singular adventure, which remained unpublished until this very day, John H. Watson, M.D., chronicled these events in a little known monograph entitled, *The Case of the Nefarious Diet Charlatans*

Once Sherlock Holmes finally unmasked this dangerous low carbohydrate diet program to the British public, these devious diet scoundrels along with Professor Moriarity fled quickly from London, and it is thought that most of them set-sail for America, where their descendants still reside. The descendants of these diet-scam artists then attempted to convince the American public of the so-called weight-loss benefits of these dangerous low carbohydrate diets. Unfortunately, like the unsuspecting Londoners, many Americans were putting their health, as well as their lives, at risk by following these dangerous, unhealthy, low carbohydrate diets. Fortunately, the first American women's magazine, *The Ladies Home Journal*, which was published in Philadelphia in 1883, exposed these diet charlatans to the American public. These nefarious scoundrels quickly disappeared from sight, until they resurfaced again in the early 1990s with a variety of new books and pamphlets touting the so-called benefits of these low-carbohydrate fad diets. It has recently been discovered that a direct descendant of Sherlock Holmes, an American physician known only as Dr. Walk, has helped to unmask these diet charlatans as being completely untruthful. He has also informed the general public about the hazards of these unhealthy diets and about the benefits of a truly healthy diet and fitness plan, utilizing a most singular program called *The Diet Fit-Step Mystery Plan*. This plan is the very cornerstone of his new monograph, entitled *The Case of the Unwanted Pounds: A Weight-Loss & Fitness Mystery*.

MODERN DAY DIET CHARLATANS

So, how do people lose weight on all of those popular low-carbohydrate, high-fat diets? For example, they say you can have bacon and eggs for breakfast, hot dogs for lunch, and a juicy steak for dinner. Sounds tempting, doesn't it? They also tell you that you can't have any, or at the very least, limited amounts of carbohydrates with each meal. For instance—no vegetables, fruits, cereals, breads, potatoes, pasta, or any whole-grain nutritious foods or desserts. Sounds unappetizing and unhealthy, doesn't it? It certainly is! And yet, over 75% of the commercially available so-called diet books work on this abnormal metabolic principle.

The simple fact is that you do lose weight, initially, on these very low carbohydrate, high fat, high-protein diets; however, most of the initial weight loss is water weight loss, due to a metabolic process called *ketosis*, which in fact is a condition found in unhealthy patients (for example: diabetes and kidney disease) not in healthy people. Once the body gets rid of the water, it starts burning fat, which is left over—which, in itself, is a good thing; however, the downside is that this abnormal process of ketosis also begins to burn the body's protein (muscle tissue). This is very dangerous. By attempting to burn protein as a source of fuel for energy, the body is actually breaking down one of its most important elements, protein, which is used to sustain life (building and repairing the body's tissues, cells and organs). The fact that a substance called ketones appears in your urine (a by-product of this abnormal process called ketosis), shows you clear evidence that your body is breaking down its muscle tissue. This is one of the reasons that fatigue and general weakness have been reported as early side effects of this completely unhealthy diet. Also, kidney and liver damage may result if too much of the body's protein is broken down from these unhealthy, high-protein, high-fat, low-carbohydrate diets. And to make matters worse, these diets are deficient in vitamins, minerals and essential nutrients.

These rapid weight loss programs (low-carbohydrate, high-fat, and high protein diets) also have the added downside of what's called "rebound weight gain." This occurs after the initial weight loss, which results from fat and protein breakdown used for energy production (fuel). The body's carbohydrate stores then become depleted because of the very low intake of carbohydrates in these diets, and thus, there is limited availability of carbohydrate to be burned as a fuel. Unfortunately, these low stores of carbohydrates are designed to be the very first type of calories to be burned as fuel in our normal metabolism.

Once your body becomes aware that it is carbohydrate depleted by exhibiting the symptoms of fatigue, malaise, muscle cramps, and decreased urine output, which occurs after the initial water loss, then your brain's control center receives stress (SOS) signals from all of the body's cells suffering from carbohydrate depletion. Once your brain's central control center receives this flood of distress messages, it immediately realizes it needs a cheaper source of fuel (refined carbohydrate and sugar) to prevent brain damage from the lack of glucose that the brain needs in order to function. Just when you're feeling exhausted and done in by this enemy low-carbohydrate diet, your hunger center sets you off on a carbohydrate binge, to counteract this lethargy you've been feeling for weeks or months. And then what happens is that your body explodes into its former overweight self, hence the term "rebound weight gain." Eventually, your sweet tooth gets satisfied, and then you resume your unhealthy diet of excess fat and refined carbohydrates. Not a pretty picture, is it?

THE CASE OF THE DIET FIT-STEP MYSTERY

This mystery case presents a series of quick and easy weight-loss and fitness clues to rid the body permanently of unwanted pounds. Weight-loss is fast, safe, effective, and easy, without all of the health risks associated with low-carbohydrate, high-fat diets. Fitness is accomplished by a simple aerobic walking program without the risks inherent to strenuous exercises.

Clue #1 presented in this weight-loss mystery is to limit your *total fat intake to 35 Grams daily* and to consume at least *35 Grams of fiber every day*. The Quick Weight-Loss Formula is a healthy, safe, and easy-to-follow diet. It consists primarily of eating low-fat, high fiber, and lean protein foods. This weight-loss plan limits your daily intake to no more than 35 grams of total fat per day and increases your consumption of fiber to 35 or more grams daily. There are no severe restrictions of any particular food group, except for foods that are high in saturated fats. Within reason, most fruits and vegetables can be eaten in unlimited quantities, with some exceptions noted below.

Clue #2 to this weight-loss and fitness mystery is an aerobic exercise walking program. *Walking for 35 minutes* six days per week boosts the weight-loss benefits of the diet plan by burning additional calories, and improving cardiovascular fitness by providing additional amounts of oxygen to the body. This plan provides you with boundless energy, while keeping you fit, and trim, without strenuous back-breaking exercises.

Clue #3 in this weight-loss and fitness plan is the addition of *strength-training exercises*. By walking with 1-2 lb. hand-held weights, for 35 minutes three days per week, you add the element of upper body strength-training and body-shaping exercises to your weight-loss and fitness mystery program. This easy plan features a unique combination of 35 minutes of aerobic exercise-walking six days per week, combined with walking for 35 minutes three days per week, using light, hand-held weights for strength-training. This combination of an aerobic exercise and strength training delivers a double-blast of calorie burning, for complete cardiovascular fitness, maximum weight-loss and complete body-shaping.

The details of these three mystery clues are explained at the end of this chapter, just as they would be in any mystery book. We will explore the characters of the innocent victims along with the guilty parties at the end of this mystery. We will also determine who the detective is, and how he/she discovers the murderer, and who his victim or victims were in this dastardly murder mystery case.

THE MYSTERY OF YOUR BODY'S METABOLISM

I. HOW YOUR BODY BURNS CALORIES (FUEL)

A. BASAL METABOLIC RATE: Just eating food burns calories! Sounds too good to be true, but it actually is a fact. Your body burns up a certain amount of calories from the foods that you eat (carbohydrate, fat and protein) and turns part of it into fuel that you need to function every day. Protein, carbohydrate and fat each burn a different amount of calories in this conversion process. If your body realizes there are not enough calories in your diet, it switches on to a slower metabolic rate in an attempt to protect you from starvation, as in times of famine—it's a natural physiologic reaction.

Unfortunately, obese people stay in the slow metabolic rate mode because they usually go on and off diets frequently, consequently it becomes difficult for them to lose weight. The metabolic rate, therefore, stays in the slow mode, because the body never knows when it will get enough food to sustain life. Then, at times when there are excess calories in their diet, weight is easily gained because their metabolism is stuck in the slow mode.

B. EXERCISE: The most important way to burn calories is by exercise. This certainly is a more efficient method of losing weight than by just relying on your body to burn calories by the sedentary process of just eating food. (Remember, just the act of eating food with no exercise whatsoever burns a certain amount of calories.)

1. Fast, quick, physical exercise such as jogging, running, tennis, basketball, racquet-ball, strenuous aerobic exercises, and race walking, burns primarily carbohydrate stores in the production of energy.

2. Slow, repetitious physical activity such as walking and swimming burns primarily fat stored in the body, which is the best type of exercise for sustained weight loss.

C. Foods That We Eat: In general, we burn almost all of the protein and carbohydrates that we eat every day. We store the remaining carbohydrates in our muscles and liver in the form of a chemical compound called glycogen. This glycogen is used for the future production of energy. The difference between the energy supplied by protein and carbohydrate in our diets and our total energy needs each day has to come from burning fats.

Weight gain actually occurs from taking in more calories in the form of dietary fats than were burned off as fuel for energy. On a low-fat diet, calories are removed from storage in fat cells and are added to the fuel mixture of protein and carbohydrate for the production of energy. This results in steady, permanent weight loss, unlike the temporary water weight loss of low-carbohydrate, high-protein diets. It's simple—*less fat taken in results in more storage fat being burned as fuel*, resulting in more fat lost from your body. More fat taken in results in more fat being stored, and less fat being burned, and lumpy, unsightly fat cells remaining!

II. How Your Body Changes Food Into Energy

A. Protein in our diet is not a significant factor in weight regulation. Almost all of the energy contained in the protein that you eat is burned as fuel for the body's metabolic process of functioning (living). Hardly any of the calories contained in dietary protein is converted into fat storage. Only 75% of the energy contained in protein can be used for your metabolic processes such as repairing the body cells, because it takes almost 25% of the energy in protein just to change it into a form that our body can use to build and repair the body's cells, tissues and organs.

B. FAT, on the other hand, is easily converted into energy. Whereas almost none of the calories contained in protein in our diets are converted into fat cells (storage), almost 95% of the dietary fat calories can be stored in fat cells when you take in excess calories of fat in your diet. In other words—**it is the fat in your diet that makes you fat!** It is not necessarily the number of calories in your diet that makes you fat, it is the number of fat calories that makes you fat.

C. CARBOHYDRATES: Before we can discuss a healthy weight loss program, we have to talk briefly about carbohydrates. Carbohydrates are the body's natural source of fuel to produce energy. One of the most important basic metabolic functions of the body is to use almost all of the carbohydrate calories you eat, as a source of fuel for energy production.

The leftover carbohydrate calories not immediately used for fuel to produce energy are stored in your liver and your muscles as a product called "glycogen," which is stored as a ready source of fuel whenever the body needs it. It is readily available and can be retrieved from the liver and muscles into the bloodstream easily, where it is quickly converted to a substance called glucose (sugar), where it then becomes available to burn as a fuel for energy production. The best part of all is that only 5 to 10% of the carbohydrate that you eat is converted as storage into fat cells. That amounts to almost 90% being available for immediate or reserve fuel for energy production, without hardly any of the carbohydrates that you eat being converted into fat. To put it simply—*complex carbohydrates in your diet will not make you fat!*

Your body expends 2½ times more energy converting dietary carbohydrate calories from your intestines into your bloodstream for immediate energy use, and then into glycogen storage in your muscles and liver, than it takes to convert fat into a source of fuel for energy production. This means that almost all of the excess fat calories that you eat are stored in fat cells, and end up staying there indefinitely. In other words a *high complex carbohydrate, low-fat diet* causes your body to work harder after each meal burning calories for energy, than does a high-fat, low-carbohydrate diet. This means that your basal metabolic rate (the rate at which your body operates all of its functions) is considerably higher on the high-carbohydrate, low-fat diet. This higher basal metabolic rate results in an additional burning of approximately 250 calories daily by the simple thermic effect of converting carbohydrates into energy.

III. How Your Body Stores Fuel

A. FAT: Fat is stored in fat cells (adipose tissue) in a ratio of four parts fat and one part water. Since there are *nine calories in each gram of fat*, it means that it takes 3500 calories to gain one pound of body fat. It therefore takes a deficit of 3500 calories to lose just one pound of fat.

Fat, unfortunately, can be stored in unlimited quantities. Normal weight individuals have almost 100,000 calories stored in fat cells. By increasing fat in the diet, combined with a sedentary lifestyle, it is quite easy to add another 50,000 to 100,000 calories in fat stores, increasing your weight 15 to 30 pounds every year. The only way to lose even one pound of body weight is to burn approximately 3500 calories. This can only be accomplished by cutting back on the amount of fat in the diet, and by increasing physical activity. Nothing else works! One of my favorite sayings to my patients when they ask me how to lose weight is: *"The only way you can lose weight is to eat less and walk more, or you can walk more and eat less!"*

B. CARBOHYDRATE: Carbohydrates that we eat are changed into a type of sugar (glucose in the bloodstream) to be used as an immediate source of fuel for the production of energy. Since only a small amount of the carbohydrates we eat is changed into immediate fuel sources, the majority of the carbohydrates consumed are changed into glycogen for storage in the liver and muscles. Remember, there are only 4 calories in each gram of carbohydrate (not 9 calories as in fat).

Glycogen is stored in the liver and muscles in a ratio of one part glycogen to four parts water (just the opposite of fat storage which is four parts fat to one part water). The liver's capacity to store glycogen is limited to approximately 500 calories and the muscles can store about 1500 calories. Muscle tissue, however, can store extra calories when you exercise so that your muscles burn energy more efficiently. When you increase your glycogen stores by 500 calories, you will gain a pound of body weight and when you decrease your glycogen stores by 500 calories, you will lose a pound of body weight. This weight, as you can see from the above ratio of glycogen to water, is mostly water weight.

NO MORE UNHEALTHY DIETS

Most men and women realize that the so-called ideal weights found in magazines and in clothing advertisements are completely unobtainable. One of the main problems with dieting is the fact that people who are on diets frequently, binge-eat far more often than non-dieters. Dieters do not eat according to whether they feel hungry, but actually eat out of the false notion that they are being good or bad. If in fact they eat a dessert that they feel "is bad for them," then frustration and anxiety sets in and they take new oaths to do better the next time. In effect then, it is not the dieter, but the diet, which is to be blamed. As Benjamin Franklin once said, *"One should eat to live, not live to eat."*

When you start limiting your food intake, neurochemicals in the brain respond as if the body were starving itself. Therefore your metabolic rate slows down so that the body does not burn food as quickly, in an attempt to conserve calories. By limiting your food intake, unfortunately this results in food cravings, which is exactly the opposite effect that you are trying to achieve. The psychological and physiological effects of dieting can sometimes be devastating. In our culture it is very easy to not like our bodies. The mirror becomes the enemy, and we feel captured in our reflection. It is only natural then, that we feel if we deprive ourselves of food, we will then be released from the prison in the mirror.

According to behavioral psychologists, children left to themselves will select a variety of foods and when they have had enough they stop eating. Adults, on the other hand, identify foods as either being good (healthy) or bad (unhealthy), and attempt, although usually not successfully, to make their selection from them. The road to normal eating is to stop listening to the myriad of advice about what to eat and start to follow your own biological and physiological needs for essential nutrients. We all know that fruits, vegetables, grains and fish are good for you; however, you must tune up your psychological and physiological metabolism in order to actually make other healthy pleasurable choices as well.

Snacking occasionally on junk food is inevitable, and as long as you do not beat yourself up over it, you will not sabotage your diet. On the other hand, if snacks are restricted permanently then your brain's neurochemical transmitters will send you into a binge-eating frenzy. Once your brain is satisfied with an occasional small self-satisfying snack or dessert, your brain's appetite control mechanism (appestat) will keep your hunger under control for longer periods of time, and this will let you concentrate on a diet that's really healthy.

The Mystery of the Diet Fit-Step Plan

Remember, you live in your body and you do not have to make drastic changes in order to feel good about yourself. The Diet Fit-Step Plan will enable you to lose as much weight as you want to in order to feel comfortable with your body. You will also develop maximum cardiovascular fitness, a firm, toned body and boundless energy on this wonderful new program. This plan was developed for my patients, who like most of you, were tired of the endless, short-lived fad diets and the myriad of strenuous exercise programs that were completely unrealistic.

The problem with most diet and exercise programs is that they are too complicated. There are too many tables to consult, too many diet meal plans to prepare and too many strenuous exercises to do. Most of these plans don't realize that everyone has a life to lead that is packed full of a hundred things to do each week. People don't really have the time to follow any type of complicated or time-consuming diet or weight-loss plans. The beauty of the Diet Fit-Step Plan is that it is designed especially for women and men who have limited amounts of time for diet and exercise, but who, on the other hand, would like a simple-easy-effective weight-loss plan that doesn't interfere with the rest of their lives. It's that simple! It's easy and effective, and it doesn't take a lot of your valuable time, and it actually works!

I originally developed this program for my patients, who, like most of you, wanted a diet and exercise plan that doesn't interfere with day-to-day living. You'll be delighted at how easy the program is, and how well it works. The Diet Fit-Step Plan is easy to follow and will help you to lose weight, keep fit and healthy. There are no complicated diet plans to follow, no diet shakes to consume or weight-loss clinics to join. This is a truly simple, easy to follow, effective weight-loss program with a minimum of time and effort on your part.

Different people respond very differently to diet and fitness programs. The mystery of *The Diet Fit-Step Plan* is that it takes all of that into consideration in the formulation of the plan. This program is designed for people of all ages and all types of body builds. It doesn't matter whether you're slightly overweight or obese, short or tall, athletic or unconditioned, young or old, muscular or flabby—this is the perfect weight-loss plan for you. This weight-loss program is not only geared towards your individual body build, but also towards your metabolic rate and your body's chemical composition. This plan will also boost your energy level and increase your metabolism as you burn-off unwanted fat calories. Give it only 21 days, and I promise you a fit, thin and trim body. You can actually *lose up to 15 pounds and 3 inches in 21 days, and easily lose those unwanted pounds.*

The Diet Fit-Step Mystery Clues

Clue 1: Diet-Step® 35/35 Plan.

The 1ˢᵗ clue consists of a diet of no more than *35 grams of total fat* and no less than *35 grams of fiber* each day. The quick weight-loss formula combines foods that are low in saturated fats and high in heart-healthy monounsaturated fats. Also, the diet limits refined, bad carbohydrates and substitutes healthy complex good carbohydrates, consisting of fruits, vegetables and whole-grain products. The Diet-Step Plan lets you lose weight at your own pace without complicated diet plans, counting calories, fad diets or starvation techniques. The plan is easy-to-follow, and quite effective for losing weight quickly and maintaining the weight that you've lost.

1. *Decrease the amount of saturated fats in your diet* (fatty meats, fatty fowl like duck and dark meat of chicken and turkey), whole dairy products including butter, margarine and hydrogenated or partially hydrogenated oils (corn, palm, safflower and other vegetable oils). These oils are also present in the form of trans-fats contained in prepared, packaged and processed foods like chips, cookies, crackers, cake mixes, frozen dinners, margarine, vegetable spreads and any and all products that contain trans fats. Limit your total fat intake to no more than 35 grams daily for good health and weight-loss. By limiting your total fat intake, you will automatically limit your intake of unhealthy saturated fats.

2. *Increase the amounts of heart-healthy monounsaturated fats with omega-3 fatty acids,* such as olive, canola oils and peanut oils, nuts and seeds, all types of beans and legumes, avocados, fish and flax seeds. Use non-fat or 1% milk, yogurt and cheeses and soy protein products. Also include the new heart healthy vegetable spreads, e.g. Promise®, Benecol®, Smart Balance®, I Can't Believe It's Not Butter® and other Trans Fat-Free spreads. These spreads should contain healthy monounsaturated fats and heart-healthy omega-3 fatty acids.

3. ***Eat no less than 35 Grams of high fiber, complex good carbohydrate foods daily****,* consisting of fruits, vegetables, nuts, beans, lentils, seeds, and whole-grain foods. Fruits and vegetables are allowed in almost unlimited quantities. These good carbohydrates have a low glycemic index, which prevents spikes in insulin levels, which cause sudden drops in blood sugar and results in fat being deposited in your fat cells. Concentrate on eating healthy whole grain breads, cereals, pasta and other whole grains such as bran, wheat germ, bulgur and whole grain rice, avocados, sweet potatoes, nuts, seeds, beans and legumes. Consume at least 35 or more grams of fiber daily for good health and weight-loss.

   Sneak in the veggies and the fruits whenever possible. Most people don't get their three servings each of fruits and vegetables daily. The way to sneak in your daily allotment of fruits and vegetables is to add them to almost any food that you order or eat that doesn't come with fruits or vegetables included. For instance, get fruit (berries, bananas, apples) on your waffles or pancakes. Add green peppers, mushrooms, onions, broccoli, or spinach to your pizza. Put salsa on your salad or sandwich. Use sliced apples, pears and grapes in your salads. Put a sliced banana on your peanut butter sandwich. Order a veggie burger instead of a meat burger. Load up any sandwich with cucumbers, tomatoes, lettuce, and sprouts. In most cases within reason, you can *eat as many fresh fruits and vegetables (raw or steamed—no butter or oils added) as you'd like to eat.* The vegetables that would be excluded from this "eat as much as you'd like list," are potatoes, corn, and beans including soybeans, avocados, and olives.

4. ***Eliminate refined, so-called bad carbohydrates*** from your diet, which include refined sugar, white flour, white rice and white pasta; processed and packaged foods; baked goods (pastries, biscuits, cookies, crackers, cakes, muffins, etc., that are made with trans-fats (hydrogenated or partially hydrogenated oils). These include all white processed grains, pastas, breads, rice, corn and white potatoes. Refined sugar causes your blood

sugar and insulin levels to peak, which in turn increases your appetite and stores unwanted fat deposits in your body.

5. The Diet Fit-Step Plan also adds ***healthy lean protein***, for increased energy, fitness and appetite control. Include beans, nuts, seeds, beans, lentils legumes, and whole-grain products. Also eat moderate amounts of other lean protein foods, consisting of low-fat dairy foods (milk, cheese, yogurt, tofu and soy), egg whites and other vegetable protein products. You can also to add low-fat lean non-vegetable protein to your diet, such as fish, poultry without the skin and very lean cuts of lamb, pork, veal and occasionally beef (small portions only with all of the fat trimmed off).

When you are on a low calorie diet, your body needs more protein for the production of energy and your body's cell maintenance. Protein is the essential nutrient responsible for the maintenance and repair of all your organs, tissues, muscles, brain and bones. All foods are sources of energy; however, protein provides a greater boost in energy levels since it is absorbed slowly and thus produces a constant source of energy.

Stay away from harmful protein. Most high-protein diets have you eating 3-4 times more protein than the recommended dietary allowance, and in most cases, the high-protein you are actually eating is the harmful, high-fat protein. These diets tax your kidneys and leach out calcium from your bones, in addition to contributing to elevated blood cholesterol, heart disease and strokes. Minimize fatty meats, fatty poultry with the skin intact and whole dairy products such as whole milk and dairy products, butter, margarine, and vegetable oils (except olive, canola and peanut oils). Even though egg yolks are high in cholesterol, they are extremely low in saturated fat. Egg yolks have gotten a lot of bad press over the years because of their high cholesterol levels; however, 3 or 4 egg yolks per week can actually be beneficial because of their high content of protein, nutrients and important antioxidants.

CLUE 2: FIT-STEP®: 35 MINUTE PLAN.

The 2ⁿᵈ clue consists of 35 minutes of an aerobic exercise walking program six days per week for an additional calorie burning power boost. Walking also produces a fresh supply of oxygen surging through your blood vessels to all of your body's tissues and cells. The Fit-Step Plan boosts the weight-loss power of the Diet-Step Plan by burning additional calories with a **35 minute aerobic exercise walking plan six days per week.** On the Fit-Step plan you will also develop maximum cardiovascular physical fitness, good health and longevity (Chapter 6).

Walking is the very best and safest aerobic exercise. Walking regularly helps your body deliver a steady supply of oxygen to all of your body's cells, tissues and organs. This increased blood supply of oxygen to your body's cells keeps your body's metabolism in perfect balance and helps you to burn extra fat calories so that you can lose weight quickly and safely. Strenuous exercises can do considerably more harm than good, as you'll see later in this mystery book.

Exercise to burn more calories than you eat. It's not necessary to join a gym or participate in aerobics classes to burn up fat. You can burn calories by just climbing the stairs, cleaning the house, riding a bike, working in the garden, or just by walking 35 minutes every day. You don't even have to work up a sweat to burn calories while exercising. Studies have proven that people who take a brisk walk for 35 minutes every day burn body fat, improve their physical fitness, and lower their blood pressure, as much as, if not even more than, people who work out at a gym three to four days per week. Even two 20-minute walks per day will give you the same fitness and fat-burning benefits as one 35 minute walk every day. A recent study from a major university showed that sedentary women, in addition to gaining weight externally, actually increased the amount of deep fat that surrounds the internal organs of the body. This increases the risk of heart disease, hypertension, and diabetes. The study also showed that moderate exercise five times per week for 30 to 40 minutes daily decreased the deep fat by more than 35% and resulted in considerable weight loss over a three-month period.

CLUE 3: BODY-SHAPING PLAN

The 3rd clue is the body-shaping plan, which adds **strength-training exercises,** to both the Diet-Step Plan and the Fit-Step Plan. By adding weight-bearing exercises to your walking program you will in effect have a *double blast of metabolic calorie burning*, by combining an aerobic exercise with strength training exercises. Strength-training also builds muscles, strengthens bones, and boosts your metabolism. This is easily accomplished by using light, hand-held weights during your 35 minute walk, three days per week. This plan, in addition to helping you lose weight, will actually sculpt and mold all of your body's muscles, which will give you a stronger and shapelier figure (Chapter 10).

There is no need to do strenuous exercises or power weight lifting in order to strengthen and shape your body. When you walk for 35 minutes using light, hand-held weights, three days per week, you will develop maximum cardiovascular fitness, increased calorie burning for additional weight-loss, and body-shaping. This addition of weight-bearing exercises strengthens your bones, builds strong muscles, and boosts your metabolic rate. These strength-training exercises are what strengthens and shapes your body's muscles and figure. This double-blast of calorie burning from the aerobic effects of walking, combined with the additional calorie-burning from the strength-training exercise, is the final clue that makes this plan so successful. The Diet Fit-Step Mystery Plan**,** will help you to slim down, shape up and look younger. *You can actually lose up to 15 pounds and 3 inches in 21 days, and finally shed those unwanted pounds.*

THE DIET FIT-STEP MYSTERY SOLVED

If you follow the clues set forth in the *Diet Fit-Step Mystery Plan* you will discover that you are in fact the *Chief Detective* in charge of the case. It's up to you to avoid getting murdered by saturated fats and a lack of exercise. The *high-fiber foods* with all of their nutrients are your secret agents, who make sure that you, the chief detective, eat a healthy diet, which is free of saturated fats and dangerous refined carbohydrates. These harmful fats including the dangerous trans-fat and refined carbohydrates can cause fat to build up in your arteries and cause heart attacks and strokes. The *complex good carbohydrates* are your loyal police staff, who also keep your body free of those dastardly fatty deposits. The *omega-3 fatty acids* found in your faithful guardians, the *monounsaturated fats*, help to protect you from cardiovascular diseases and the degenerative diseases of aging, including many forms of cancer. These monounsaturated allies also prevent the buildup of fatty deposits in your arteries by gunning down the dangerous saturated fats that are your mortal enemies. Your other secret agent, *lean protein*, will keep your metabolism working smoothly and all of your body's organs functioning properly.

And last but not least, your trusted side-kick, *Detective Walk*, keeps you safe from the deadly consequences of a sedentary lifestyle. Detective Walk helps you to stay fit and healthy, despite all of the deadly criminals out there who would love to see you sit still and then die of a heart attack, high blood pressure, a stroke, a neurological disease, or some form of cancer. Also, Detective Walk's first sergeant, who specializes in strength-training, will keep your bones and muscles strong and your body in great shape. Detective Walk has the uncanny ability to keep you healthy and fit in spite of yourself, as long as you follow his daily exercise walking routine and stay away from a sedentary lifestyle and dangerous strenuous exercises. These nefarious criminals (saturated fats, trans-fats, refined carbohydrates, fatty protein, sedentary lifestyle and strenuous exercises) will all be arrested, prosecuted, and incarcerated by the legal-health system, because of the testimony of Detective Walk and his secret agents. And rest assured that no fancy criminal lawyer will ever get these dangerous criminals off on any of these charges. They will serve time for their deadly dietary and evil sedentary discretions.

20 The Case of the Unwanted Pounds

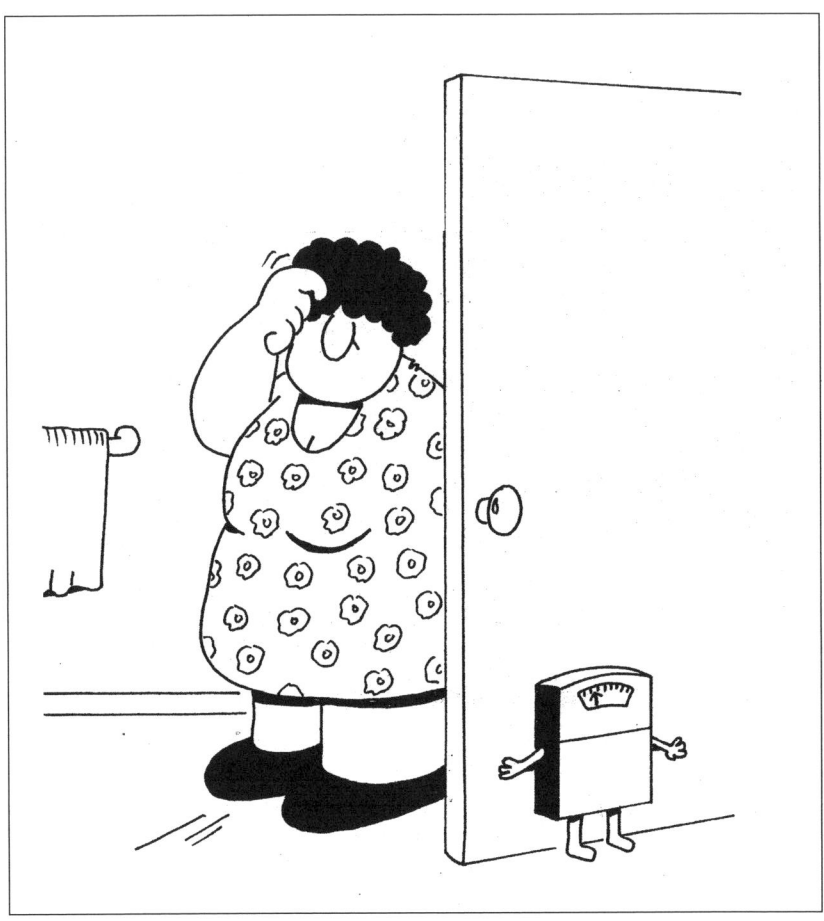

"Oh no, not another diet again."

2

21-Day Quick Weight-Loss Plan

The **Diet Fit-Step Mystery Plan** consists of eating 35 grams of fat and 35 grams of fiber daily, combined with 35 minutes of walking six days per week. Weight loss is fast and easy, and what's more, it's permanent. There is no rebound weight gain, no food cravings, no starvation techniques, no liquid protein drinks and no diet pills. And no unhealthy low-carb diets to follow, where you end up stuffing your face with meat, eggs, cheese, butter, cream, bacon, fat and more fat, until you and your arteries are ready to explode. The mystery of the Diet Fit-Step Plan is that you'll easily get rid of those unwanted pounds quickly and permanently.

The Diet Fit-Step Plan is specifically designed for people of all ages, all shapes, all sizes and all weights. The quick weight loss plan is easy to follow and works quickly to shed all of the extra unwanted pounds that you want to lose. Remember to walk for 35 minutes six days per week which is discussed in more detail in Chapter 6. This easy plan is essentially a diet that is high in fiber, complex carbohydrates and lean protein. This diet limits your intake of saturated fats, cholesterol, refined carbohydrates and sugars, and salt, caffeine and alcohol. When combined with a 35-minute walk 6 days per week, it is the only diet that has been proven to be effective in permanent weight loss, weight control, fitness and good health.

By limiting the total grams of fat to 35 grams daily, we eliminate many high fat calories that add extra weight and can block your arteries with saturated fat and cholesterol. Remember that *each gram of fat contains 9 calories compared to 4 calories each from protein and carbohydrates.* The high fiber content (35 grams per day) in this diet also provides a built-in mechanism against gaining weight and developing many degenerative diseases of aging. See the Fat & Fiber Counter in the Appendix, in order to count the number of grams of fat and fiber in your diet. You can actually lose up to 15 pounds and 3 inches in only 21 days, as you easily get rid of those unwanted pounds on the Diet Fit-Step Plan.

QUICK WEIGHT LOSS FORMULA

1. Eat no more than 35 Grams of Total Fat Daily (concentrate on heart-healthy fats and reduce saturated fats)

2. Eat no less than 35 Grams of Fiber daily.

3. Within reason, you can eat as many fruits and raw or steamed vegetables (no added butter or oils), as you'd like. The only exceptions are potatoes, corn, and beans including soybeans, avocados or olives.

4. Do not eat refined or processed foods (sugar, white flour, and white rice). Do not eat packaged or commercially baked goods made with hydrogenated or partially hydrogenated oils.

5. Limit salt, caffeine and alcohol.

6. Drink at least six 8 oz. glasses of water daily.

7. Walk 35 minutes, six days per week.

DIET-STEP®: 35/35 MEAL PLANS

The basic diet is divided into easy to follow meal plans. Each of these daily diet meal plans has already been formulated to contain 35 grams of total fat and 35 grams fiber per day, without your having to add up the number of grams of fat and fiber.

Once you've completed the first few weeks of your diet, these basic Diet-Step Meal Plans will become an automatic part of your everyday schedule. The diet is extremely easy to follow. Once you've become comfortable with the basic meal plans, you can then start to formulate your own individual meals by eating no more than 35 grams of total fat and no less than 35 grams of fiber daily. Consult the Fat and Fiber Counter in the Appendix, and then you can mix and match any individual meal that you'd like.

There is such a variety of foods included in this 35/35 diet that your taste buds will never tire of this healthful, nutritious, palatable diet program. By varying the foods in your diet, there are never any hunger pangs or food cravings. The Fat & Fiber Counter in the Appendix will allow you to choose any foods that you want. Remember that the Diet-Step Plan, in addition to controlling your weight, will add years to your life by providing essential, healthy nutrients, antioxidants, phyto-nutrients, vitamins and minerals, which eliminate harmful free-radical components from your body. This is a diet and exercise plan for fitness and health as well as for weight loss and body-shaping.

After you have reached your ideal weight on this easy diet program, you will never again have to worry about rebound weight gain. The Diet-Step: 35/35 plan enables you to lose weight quickly utilizing only these basic sample menu plans during your initial weight-loss program, or by following any of the optional meal plans, which are listed at the end of the basic weekly meal plans. Also, you can choose any combination of meals (breakfast, lunch and dinner) containing 35 grams of fat and 35 grams of fiber found in the Fat and Fiber Counter. You will lose weight quickly and safely on the Diet-Step: 35/35 Plan.

	MONDAY
BREAKFAST	1 whole medium orange or ½ grapefruit ¾ cup cold whole grain or bran cereal with ½ cup any fresh fruit & ½ cup non-fat milk 1-2 cups coffee or tea (non-fat milk and artificial sweetener) 8 oz. glass water
LUNCH	1 cup soup (any type except cream based) – the more vegetables and beans, the better 1 whole wheat or multi-grain veggie sandwich with lettuce, tomatoes, sprouts, cucumber, carrots or any leafy green vegetable. Add Dijon mustard and sliced pickles. 1 glass decaffeinated sugar-free (coffee, tea, or soda) 8 oz. glass water
SNACK	1 medium orange or tangerine or handful of almonds or walnuts 8 oz. glass water
DINNER	Vegetable platter (broccoli, asparagus, squash, cauliflower, baked beans, carrots, green beans, spinach, mushrooms, stewed tomatoes, cauliflower) – choose any 4 (½ cup each) 1 whole-wheat dinner roll 4 oz. red wine or 12 oz. light beer 8 oz. glass water
SNACK	½ cup raisins with 2 tbs. nuts (almonds, pecans or walnuts) *-or-* 1 cup mixed fresh fruit (strawberries, blueberries, blackberries purple grapes, bananas, etc.) *-or-* 1 high fiber, low-fat oat and chocolate bar with ½ glass skim milk 8 oz. glass water

Total grams fat: 34.8 Total grams fiber: 35.2
WALK 35 MINUTES

TUESDAY

BREAKFAST
¾ cup cooked whole grain (oatmeal) or bran cereal with raisins (¼ cup) or any fresh fruit, cinnamon, ½ cup non-fat milk

1 medium orange or 1 medium tangerine

1-2 cups coffee or tea (non-fat milk, artificial sweetener)

8 oz. glass water

LUNCH
1 slice pizza (tomato only or light cheese), topped with your choice of green peppers, mushrooms, onions, garlic, etc.

1 large tossed salad with non-fat dressing

12 oz. diet drink of your choice (decaffeinated and sugar-free)

8 oz. glass water

SNACK
1 medium apple, pear, peach or nectarine and handful cashews

8 oz. glass water

DINNER
3 oz. baked eggplant or zucchini casserole parmesan baked with 1 tsp. olive oil and lightly breaded with whole wheat breading or 2 crumbled whole wheat crackers

1 cup steamed veggies (cauliflower, broccoli, spinach, etc.)

1 whole wheat roll

4 oz. tomato or vegetable juice

8 oz. glass water

SNACK
½ cantaloupe or melon with ½ cup blueberries, strawberries or raspberries *-or-* 1 piece of fresh fruit (banana, pear, apple, peach, plum, orange or nectarine)

8 oz. glass water

Total grams fat: 35.5 Total grams fiber: 34.5
WALK 35 MINUTES

WEDNESDAY

BREAKFAST
1 slice whole wheat bread or whole wheat English muffin non-fat whipped/diet margarine without trans-fats or 1 tsp. jelly)

1 whole medium orange or 1 cup mixed berries

1-2 cups coffee or tea (artificial sweetener & non-fat milk)

8 oz. glass water

LUNCH
1 cup soup (vegetable, tomato, lentil, bean, pea, celery, minestrone, consommé, chicken noodle/rice, Manhattan clam chowder – no creamed or pureed soups) and 2-3 whole-wheat crackers.

Low-fat peanut butter and jelly sandwich on whole wheat muffin

1 cup decaffeinated sugar free (coffee, tea or diet soda)

8 oz. glass water

SNACK
Small box raisins and handful of walnuts

8 oz. glass water

DINNER
Tossed salad (lettuce, tomato, cucumber, carrots, celery) with lemon and/or 1 tsp olive oil and dash of vinegar dressing or 1 tsp. non-fat dressing

3 oz. whole-wheat pasta primavera (fresh veggies and ½ cup marinara sauce with or without mushrooms and garlic) Add small amount Parmesan cheese

1 whole wheat dinner roll

4 oz. red wine or 12 oz. light beer

8 oz. glass water

SNACK
2 cups unbuttered, unsalted popcorn (hot air popcorn popper without oil)

-or- 1 cup mixed fruits (berries, purple grapes, bananas)

8 oz. glass water

Total grams of fat: 35.1 Total grams of fiber: 34.8
WALK 35 MINUTES

THURSDAY

BREAKFAST
4 medium dried or stewed prunes or ½ cantaloupe or honeydew melon or 1 cup any fresh fruit
1 slice whole or cracked wheat bread (½ teaspoon whipped/diet oil-free margarine or 1 tsp. jelly)
1-2 cups coffee or tea (artificial sweetener and non-fat milk)
8 oz. glass water

LUNCH
1 cup fresh fruit salad on bed of lettuce with ½ cup low-fat cottage cheese and 2 whole-wheat crackers *-or-*
1 small chef salad with turkey (2 slices) and low-fat cheese (1 slice) only; use lemon, vinegar or 1 tsp. non-fat dressing
1 cup decaffeinated sugar free (coffee, tea or diet soda)
8 oz. glass water

SNACK
1 medium pear *-or-* handful walnuts or almonds
8 oz. glass water

DINNER
Large tossed salad (lettuce, tomato, celery, carrots, cucumber), with non-fat dressing
3 oz. broiled or baked chicken breast, skin removed; add seasoning (paprika, garlic, pepper, etc.)
½ cup brown long whole grain rice; or ½ cup frozen corn or (1) small ear whole kernel corn (no butter, margarine, or salt)
1 cup steamed veggies (broccoli or spinach)
4 oz. tomato or vegetable juice
8 oz. glass water

SNACK
⅛ slice angel food cake with non-fat whipped cream and sliced fruit or berries
1 8 oz. glass decaffeinated tea or soda (sugar free) *-or-*
½ cup low-fat frozen yogurt or a high fiber, low-fat cereal bar
8 oz. glass water

Total grams fat: 35.4 Total grams fiber: 35.3
WALK 35 MINUTES

FRIDAY

BREAKFAST
½ medium grapefruit or 1 medium orange

¾ cup cooked or cold whole grain (bran type) unsweetened cereal with ½ cup non-fat milk, ½ medium banana or 2 dozen raisins (½ oz.)

1-2 cups coffee or tea (artificial sweetener and non-fat milk)

8 oz. glass water

LUNCH
3 oz. (½ cup) tuna or chicken salad stuffed in whole-wheat pita bread (1 tsp. fat-free mayonnaise), with lettuce, tomato and cucumber. Use tuna packed in water.

1 cup decaffeinated sugar-free (coffee, tea or diet soda)

8 oz. glass water

SNACK
1 medium peach or banana and handful Brazil nuts

8 oz. glass water

DINNER
Large tossed salad with non-fat dressing (lettuce, tomato, celery, carrot, cucumber)

3 oz. baked or broiled fish (flounder, salmon, haddock, halibut, cod, sole, bass, bluefish, perch, trout) with lemon

1 medium baked potato or baked yam including skin (no butter, margarine or sour cream)

1 cup steamed vegetables (your choice)

4 oz. red wine or 12 oz. light beer

8 oz. glass water

SNACK
2 small unsalted, whole wheat pretzels or one medium soft pretzel (Superpretzel®) with or without mustard

-or- ¾ cup non-fat yogurt or low-fat fruit cottage cheese with 2 tsp. wheat germ or Miller's bran

8 oz. glass water

Total grams of fat: 35.0 Total grams of fiber: 34.6
WALK 35 MINUTES

SATURDAY

BREAKFAST

2 eggs (egg white or artificial egg omelet) with tomato, green peppers, onions and any non-fat cheese; or 1 poached or fried egg (non-fat, oil-free margarine – soft type

1 small fresh mango, kiwi, or guava

1 slice whole wheat, rye or pumpernickel bread with all fruit jam (1 T)

1- 2 cups coffee (non-fat milk, artificial sweetener)

8 oz. glass water

LUNCH

1 cup soup any type except creamed – the more veggies and beans the better

Large tossed salad with ½ tsp. olive oil & vinegar or non-fat dressing

2 whole-wheat crackers

Diet drink of your choice (decaffeinated and sugar-free)

8 oz. glass water

SNACK

Any fruit or handful of walnuts or cashews –*or*– 1 baked apple (artificial sweetener) and cinnamon and raisins

8 oz. glass water

DINNER

3 oz. veal (lean) scaloppini or chicken (white meat without skin) cacciatore (baked with tomatoes, onions, peppers, mushrooms and garlic – your choice)

1 small baked or sweet potato with skin (no butter or sour cream)

1 slice whole wheat bread or roll

4 oz. tomato or vegetable juice

8 oz. glass water

SNACK

1 cup mixed fruit (berries, bananas, peach, grapes, kiwi, etc.)

–*or*– ½ cup of low-fat frozen yogurt

8 oz. glass water

Total grams fat: 34.7 Total grams fiber: 34.7
WALK 35 MINUTES

SUNDAY

BREAKFAST
2 small whole grain pancakes topped with fresh fruit or sugar-free syrup

1 small nectarine or tangerine

1-2 cups coffee or tea (non-fat milk, artificial sweetener)

8 oz. glass water

LUNCH
Nicoise salad: tuna (dry), tomato, ½ sliced hard boiled egg, (3) black olives, (1) anchovy, onion, bell pepper, radish and celery (balsamic vinaigrette dressing on the side – just a few fork-fulls)

Diet drink of your choice (decaffeinated and sugar-free)

8 oz. glass water

SNACK
1 small box raisins or ½ cup grapes (purple or green) with 6 almonds

8 oz. glass water

DINNER
3 oz. sirloin steak (lean) with grilled onions, mushrooms, garlic, peppers – your choice

1 medium baked potato or sweet potato with skin (no butter or sour cream)

1 cup steamed vegetables – your choice

4 oz. red wine or 12 oz. light beer

8 oz. glass water

SNACK
¾ cup sugar-free, fat-free ice cream *-or-* sugar-free jello with non-fat whipped cream *-or-* high fiber, low-fat, chocolate and oat bar

8 oz. glass water

Total grams fat: 34.8 Total grams fiber: 35.1
REST!

DIET FIT-STEP'S MYSTERY CLUES

1. The above diet plans have all been pre-calculated to contain no more than 35 grams of total fat and no less than 35 grams of fiber per day. To formulate your own combination of foods, just check the values in the **Fat & Fiber Counter** (APPENDIX) and mix and match any foods for any meals that you like. Remember to use no more than 35 grams of total fat and no less than 35 grams of fiber each day.

2. One of the most important parts of the ***Diet-Step: Quick Weight-Loss Plan*** is to keep the total fat content to no more than 35 grams daily and to concentrate on heart-healthy fats and limit saturated fats. Not only does this accelerate your weight loss, but you decrease your risk of heart attacks and strokes by reducing your blood cholesterol levels. By limiting your total fat to 35 grams daily, you in effect limit your intake of saturated fats, dietary cholesterol and trans-fatty acids—all of which can significantly raise your blood cholesterol to dangerous levels. *According to the American Heart Association, for every 1% drop in blood cholesterol, your risk of a heart attack drops 2%. Pretty impressive!*

    A. You will notice that it is not necessary to count and record the grams of cholesterol with each meal. They are listed in the Fat & Fiber Counter for your own information. The American Heart Association usually recommends no more than **300 mg. per day of dietary cholesterol**. However, by limiting your total fat intake to 35 grams/day, you will be automatically limiting your total intake of cholesterol. There are a few exceptions that we'll discuss later; for example, shell fish, which is high in cholesterol, is not high in total grams of fat. Other fatty fishes like salmon, tuna, mackerel, herring, sardines and pompano, contain high amounts of **omega-3 fatty acids** which can significantly reduce your risk of heart disease. These 3-omega fatty acids are known as the heart-healthy fats.

B. It's the **saturated fats** that you have to concentrate on eliminating from your diet, so that you'll have more room for the heart-healthy monounsaturated good fats. You will also notice a column in the Fat & Fiber Counter (Appendix) marked "Saturated Fats." These are the dietary fats that come from animal sources. These saturated fats are dangerous and can block the arteries in your heart, brain and legs. This blockage can lead to heart attacks, strokes and vascular disease. The American Heart Association recommends limiting saturated fats in your diet to a maximum of 15-20 grams daily. However, it is not necessary to count the grams of saturated fat on the Diet-Step Plan. By limiting the total grams of fat to 35 grams daily, your intake of saturated fats will be far below the recommended values. Limit meat (beef, pork, veal) intake to no more than (2) small servings per week since meat is extremely high in saturated fats.

C. Heart-healthy fats include: avocados, beans and legumes, fish, seeds and nuts (especially walnuts, almonds, cashews, and flax seeds), and certain oils (ex. olive, canola, and peanut oils). While these foods have a high total fat content, they are very low in saturated fats. They are also high in **monounsaturated fats**, which have been proven to be heart-protective. These foods can actually help to lower blood cholesterol and thereby reduce your risk of heart attacks. Nuts and seeds also contain many important vitamins and minerals, for example, selenium, which has been proven to be a potent cancer fighter. These good fats have to be limited to some extent on the quick weight loss diet, since they are usually high in total fat content, and you can't exceed 35 grams of total fat daily. However, you will be able to add more of these good fats to your diet after you've lost your first 15 pounds in 21 days.

3. An equally important factor in this diet is the **35 grams of dietary fiber** that you will be eating every day. Since fiber is primarily plant based, you will be eating lots of soluble and insoluble fiber (at least 35 grams), which also helps to reduce your cholesterol in addition to reducing your appetite. These high fiber plants also contain numerous beneficial compounds including phyto-nutrients, antioxidants, flavinoids, B & C vitamins, minerals, beta and other carotenoids and folic acid, among others. All of these compounds help to fight heart disease, cancer and many other degenerative diseases.

   A. Enjoy at least **2-3 servings from the fruit group and 2-3 servings from the vegetable group** each day which helps to control your appetite on the Diet-Step plan. For a wide variety of nutrients, choose fruits and vegetables in a rainbow of colors. As you'll see in Chapter 3, these high-fiber fruits and vegetables contain many disease fighting phyto-nutrients, vitamins and minerals. In most cases within reason, you can *eat as many fresh fruits and vegetables (raw or steamed—no butter or oils added) as you'd like to eat.* The vegetables that would be excluded from this "eat as much as you'd like" list are potatoes, corn, and beans including soybeans, avocados, and olives.

   B. Choose from an array of **high-fiber, nutritious, complex carbohydrates** that fill you up without filling you out. These foods provide high-octane fuel to power you through the day and keep you energized for physical activity. The following foods are excellent sources of fiber: barley, oats, bran, wheat germ, bulgur and brown rice; beans, peas and lentils; whole-grain breads and pastas; and most fruits and vegetables including apples, broccoli, Brussels sprouts, berries, cabbage, carrots, grapefruit, oranges, pears, plums, prunes, raisins and spinach, among others (see Fat & Fiber Counter in the Appendix).

   C. Remember to **eliminate all refined carbohydrates foods** (sugar, flour and rice) and **packaged and processed foods** and commercially **baked goods.**

4. It's important to eat a moderate amount of **lean protein** on the Diet-Step weight loss plan for proper nutrition and to help you lose weight. Eat more fish, poultry (white meat without the skin), very lean meats, egg whites, non-fat dairy and soy products, whole-grain foods, nuts, seeds and all types of beans. Lean protein is essential for proper nutrition and metabolism. Protein helps to heal, repair and maintain all of your body's cells and to regulate your basal metabolic rate.

5. Also limit the amount of **salt** (which can cause fluid retention and can lead to hypertension), and **caffeine** (which can stimulate your appetite and cause anxiety, palpitations and even high blood pressure), and also **alcohol** (which adds additional calories to your diet, so limit alcoholic drinks to 4 ounces red wine or 12 ounces light beer) 3 to 4 times per week. Excess amounts of salt and caffeine in your diet can raise your blood pressure and cause heart rhythm abnormalities. Both salt and caffeine can also actually increase your appetite. Excessive alcohol intake can add unwanted calories to your diet (7 calories per gram) and could possibly damage your liver. However, it has been shown in several medical studies that 4 ounces of red wine daily can be a heart-healthy addition to your diet, since it contains a powerful antioxidant called *resveratrol*.

6. Also remember to drink at least **six, 8 oz. glasses of water daily.** Water fills you up so that your appetite is decreased, especially if you drink 8 oz. of water before your meals. Also, water is necessary for all of your body's metabolic functions to work properly, including maintaining the electrolytes in your blood at a proper balance. An adequate amount of water in your diet also contributes to proper kidney function. Drink water before and during your meal. Water fills you up and decreases your hunger control's appetite center in the brain. You'll naturally eat less food with each meal and feel quite satisfied when you're finished eating. Water is also essential to keeping your metabolism running smoothly and in keeping all of your blood's components in perfect balance. Water also

keeps you well hydrated and controls your appetite, because being well-hydrated prevents spikes in blood insulin levels that cause your blood sugar to drop, which subsequently increases your appetite for high sugar bad carbohydrates.

7. **Avoid soft drinks.** Sweetened soft drinks contain loads of sugar and calories. In addition to sodas, this includes sweetened iced teas, fat-laden calories in coffee drinks such as lattes and cappuccinos, and juices that contain little or no fruit, but lots of sugar. Stay away from the so-called energy drinks, which contain high amounts of sugar and caffeine. These drinks are unhealthy and the energy that they produce initially is from the initial shot of caffeine and glucose absorbed into the bloodstream. These drinks cause unhealthy spikes in both blood sugar and blood insulin, and the high caffeine content of these drinks can be dehydrating. Be sure to choose diet sodas and teas. Switch to fat-free coffee drinks without sugar. Choose 100% fruit juices and 100% vegetable juices. Drink lots of water, seltzer, and fat-free milk.

8. Don't forget to **walk 35 minutes six days per week on the Fit-Step Plan.** When you combine the Diet-Step: 35 Grams Fat/35 Grams Fiber Plan with the Fit-Step: 35 Minute Walking Plan you have the **Diet Fit-Step Plan.**

9. **Don't skip breakfast.** Studies have proved that people who eat a healthy breakfast every day are the most successful dieters. A healthy breakfast consisting of a whole-grain, high-fiber cereal topped with fruit and skim milk is a great way to start the day. A hard-boiled egg or an egg fried in a small amount of olive oil on a slice of toasted whole-wheat bread makes a great lean protein start for your day. A slice of whole-wheat bread topped with a Tbs. of all-fruit jelly and/or peanut butter is an appetite-satisfying breakfast. People who regularly eat a healthy breakfast don't get hungry for midmorning snacks of doughnuts or muffins. Your body's appetite control mechanism stays in check for longer periods of time, without any spikes in blood sugar or blood insulin levels. And besides, a nutritious

breakfast causes your body to burn fat more efficiently and starts your diet-day off perfectly.

10. **Eat more frequently.** Small frequent meals keep your body fueled throughout the day and prevent you from overeating at any particular time of day or night. Small meals with lean protein and high fiber added keep your appetite satisfied for hours without any hunger pangs. Adding the lean protein to these small, frequent meals increases your energy level. If you skip breakfast or lunch, your metabolism slows down, causing a spike in insulin levels when you finally eat. This makes it harder for your body to burn fat efficiently. This results in weight gain, not weight loss. This type of small, frequent meal eating helps you to condition yourself to keeping portion sizes small when you eat at home or at a restaurant.

11. When you start to formulate your own meal combinations of 35 grams fat/35 grams fiber, you should keep a **daily record of the total grams of fat and the total grams of fiber** that you eat at each meal. Make sure that the total for each day adds up to no more than 35 grams of total fat and no less than 35 grams of fiber. You can use 3 x 5 index cards to keep your record for each individual meal, and then you'll be able to review them anytime for future use. You can also record your meal plans on your computer or on any hand-held electronic device or smart phone. Choose any method that's easy, convenient and fun for you. You will lose weight quickly and easily on the *Diet-Step Plan* without worrying about rebound weight gain.

12. **You can lose up to 15 lbs. & 3 inches in only 21 days, and re-shape your body, as you easily get rid of those unwanted pounds**. It is likely that your weight-loss will taper-off very slightly after the first 21 days; however, you will still be able to lose approximately 3 to 3½ pounds and ¼ to ½ inch per week as your body's metabolism adjusts to the Diet Fit-Step weight-loss plan. The weight you lose will stay lost forever.

35 GRAMS FAT/35 GRAMS FIBER OPTIONAL MEAL PLANS

The following lists are a variety of 35 Grams Fat/35 Grams Fiber options for your meal plans. Each meal (breakfast, lunch or dinner) has already been pre-calculated to add up to approximately ⅓ of the allotted fat and fiber grams for each day. In other words, when you combine any 3 meals (breakfast, lunch & dinner), you'll have the total allotted 35 grams fat/35 grams fiber for any given day

DIET-STEP®: BREAKFAST OPTIONS

- 1 fried egg with non-fat spray and two small veggie non-fat sausages or two slices non-fat turkey bacon
- 1 fried egg with non-fat spray and 1 slice whole wheat bread and 1 tsp. all-fruit jam
- 1 non-fat waffle with fresh fruit topping
- Two small whole wheat or buckwheat pancakes made with egg substitute topped with fresh fruit and/or sugar free syrup
- 1 poached egg with 1 slice whole wheat toast and 1 tsp. all-fruit jam
- ½ cup low-fat granola with ½ cup blueberries and strawberries
- 1 scooped-out whole wheat bagel with 1 slice unsalted smoked salmon (nova lox), with non-fat cream cheese, tomato and onion
- 1 cup cold bran-type or whole wheat cereal with ½ cup any fresh fruit
- 2 egg whites or egg substitute omelet with 1 slice low-fat (skim milk) cheese, tomato, onions, green peppers, mushrooms (any or all)
- 1 cup cooked oatmeal or wheatena with cinnamon and ¼ cup raisins
- 1 cup fat-free yogurt with fresh fruit and 1T wheat germ

- 1 scrambled egg with non-fat spray and oat bran or whole wheat English muffin with 1 tsp. all-fruit jelly
- 1 toasted small whole wheat bagel with 1 tsp. non-fat cream cheese
- 1 slice cinnamon French toast with egg substitute and whole wheat bread

Diet-Step®: Lunch Options

- 1 whole-wheat bun with two slices reduced-fat turkey breast, with lettuce, tomato, mustard or 1 tsp. non-fat mayonnaise
- 1 cup Chinese greens with 6 medium grilled shrimp and garlic with 1 cup brown rice
- 1 non-fat cream cheese (2T) and jelly (2T) sandwich on whole wheat bread
- 1 whole-wheat bagel scooped out with 2 slices low-fat cheese, grilled with tomato and Dijon mustard or 1 tsp non-fat mayonnaise
- 1 whole wheat sandwich with two slices skim milk cheese (alpine lace) or other low-fat cheese, with lettuce, tomato, shredded carrots and sprouts, with mustard or 1 tsp. non-fat mayonnaise
- 1 small can fat-free baked beans, 1 non-fat beef hot dog or turkey dog on whole wheat bun with sauerkraut, relish and mustard and small side salad with 1 tsp non-fat dressing
- 2T non-fat cream cheese sandwich on whole wheat bread with sprouts, tomato, cucumber and lettuce; 1 medium order steamed mussels or clams (12) with ½ cup marinara sauce with 1 small whole wheat roll
- 1 whole-wheat bagel scooped out with one slice smoked salmon (nova lox) with tomato, onion and lettuce
- 1 medium whole wheat pita pocket with grilled chicken breast (3 oz) and 1 tsp. non-fat mayonnaise with lettuce, tomato, celery and cucumber

- 1T reduced-fat peanut butter & 1T jelly sandwich whole wheat bread
- 1 soft corn tortilla with ⅓ cup fat-free refried beans with shredded low-fat cheese, lettuce, tomato and salsa
- ½ veggie hoagie (tomatoes, lettuce, olives, peppers, onions, cucumbers, carrots, sprouts-your choice) with roll scooped out leaving only shell of Italian roll
- 1 medium whole wheat pita pocket with tuna (3 oz) packed in water with lettuce, tomato, cucumber, sprouts and 1 tsp. Dijon mustard or 1 tsp. non-fat mayonnaise
- 1 veggie burger on whole wheat bread or bun with lettuce, tomato, onion & ketchup
- 1 cup soup (minestrone, lentil, split pea or any vegetable or bean-based soup) with one small whole-wheat roll
- 1 can (3 oz) sardines (drain oil) on whole wheat bread or pita with tomato, lettuce and onion
- spinach salad with 1 oz low-fat blue cheese, ½ oz. chopped walnuts, sliced apples, cherry tomatoes, cucumbers, in 1T dressing made with mustard, lemon and 1 tsp olive oil
- panini sandwich toasted on scooped-out Italian or French roll with tomato, low-fat mozzarella cheese, basil and lettuce
- Nicoise salad with mixed greens, tuna, string beans, tomato, anchovies, ½ sliced hardboiled egg, olives, radishes, celery, onions and bell pepper with mustard vinaigrette dressing on on the side (dip fork in dressing sparingly) and one scooped out French roll
- goat cheese salad with reduced-fat goat cheese, mixed greens, tomato, olives, bell peppers, cucumber, celery, with mustard vinaigrette dressing on the side (dip fork in dressing sparingly) and one scooped-out French roll

DIET-STEP®: DINNER OPTIONS

- 2 soft tacos with non-fat refried beans, lettuce, tomato, onion, grated non-fat cheese with 3 oz. sliced grilled chicken and salsa
- 3 oz broiled or baked cod, halibut, mackerel or sole with grilled onions, peppers, mushrooms and tomatoes, with lemon, wine and seasonings, small whole wheat dinner roll and tossed salad
- 1 cup spinach fettuccini with fresh vegetables and ½ cup tomato or marinara sauce and large tossed salad (see above)
- chicken Caesar salad with lettuce, tomato, chopped celery, cucumber and with 3 oz grilled chicken breast and non-fat parmesan cheese and 1T fat-free Caesar dressing
- 1 cup whole wheat spaghetti with 12 clams or mussels, garlic, ⅓ cup white wine, 1 tsp olive oil and seasoning and large tossed salad (see above)
- 1 grilled 3 oz lean hamburger on whole wheat roll with lettuce, tomato, onion and ketchup and 1 small white potato made into oven-baked French fries (slice into fries, spray nonstick pan with non-fat spray and bake on 400 degrees until crisp)
- 1 small can of sardines (drain oil) or tuna packed in water in large tossed salad of lettuce or romaine, tomato, cucumber, pepper, onion, sprouts, carrots and olives and 1 tsp non-fat dressing or mustard-vinaigrette dressing
- 1 slice pizza (tomato, or with light cheese and tomato) topped with veggies of your choice and a side salad with 1 tsp non-fat dressing
- 3 oz lean roast beef with horseradish and small baked potato or yam with skin, 1 cup steamed veggies and small whole wheat roll

- 1 cup low-fat macaroni and cheese with 1 cup zucchini, diced tomatoes, onions and garlic and an ear of corn or a small sweet potato and steamed fresh carrots (½ cup)
- 6 medium cooked peeled shrimp with cocktail sauce and small ear of corn and 1 cup steamed asparagus, broccoli or spinach
- 3 oz. grilled salmon steak or salmon fillet with tomatoes, onions, peppers and garlic and small baked potato or yam and 1 cup steamed vegetable (your choice)
- 2 small lamb chops (trim fat) with 2 tsp. mint jelly and whole broiled tomato with 1 small baked sweet potato and tossed salad (see above)

KEEPING YOUR HEART HEALTHY THROUGH GOOD NUTRITION AND EXERCISE

You can do a lot to reduce your risk of heart disease by eating right and exercising. Here are some tips on what to eat and what to stay away from. At the end, you will find some advice on exercise. This should start you on your way to a healthier heart.

BREADS, CEREALS, RICE, AND PASTA: SIX OR MORE SERVINGS PER DAY

Foods to eat	Foods to avoid
- Breads with at least 2 grams of fiber per serving (examples: whole grain bread, English muffins, bagels, buns, corn and flour tortillas) - Oat, wheat, corn, and multigrain cereals with at least 5 grams of fiber per serving - Whole wheat pasta - Brown rice - Low-fat animal crackers, graham crackers, soda crackers, bread sticks, melba toast, and other crackers that have all of the following: less than 2 grams of fat per serving; at least 1 gram of fiber per serving; no hydrogenated oil - Homemade baked goods made with unsaturated oil, skim or 1 percent milk, and egg substitute (examples: quick breads, biscuits, cornbread, muffins, bran muffins, pancakes, waffles)	- Breads with fat, butter, or eggs listed as one of the first ingredients (examples: croissants, tortillas made with added fats) - Granola made with partially hydrogenated oil - White pasta - White rice - High-fat crackers and those made with partially hydrogenated oil - Commercially baked pastries, biscuits

Vegetables:
At least three to five servings per day

Foods to eat	Foods to avoid
• Fresh or frozen vegetables without added fat or salt • Vegetables stir fried with small amounts of unsaturated oil	• Vegetables fried or cooked with butter, cheese, or cream sauce

Fruits: 2 cups per day
(about two regular-sized pieces of fruit)

Foods to eat	Foods to avoid
• A variety of fruits; all fruits are allowed. Limit dried fruit to ½ cup.	

Nuts and seeds, including olives and avocados:
½ cup per day most days

Foods to eat	Foods to avoid
• Seeds and nuts, including avocados, olives, natural peanut butter (no more than 2 tablespoons per day)	• Coconut, peanut butter made with partially hydrogenated oil

Dairy products and dairy substitutes: three servings (each 1 cup) per day	
Foods to eat	*Foods to avoid*
• Skim milk, thick skim milk, 1 percent milk, buttermilk • Soy or rice drinks • Low-fat cheese with less than 3 grams of fat per serving, including natural cheese, processed cheese, and nondairy cheese such as soy cheese • Low-fat, nonfat, and dry-curd cottage cheese with less than 2 percent fat • Low-fat or nonfat coffee creamer and sour cream (read the label, and avoid if sugar is one of the first three ingredients)	• Whole milk, 2 percent milk • Yogurt and yogurt drinks made with whole milk • Regular cheeses (examples: American, blue, Brie, cheddar, Colby, Edam, Monterey Jack, part-skim mozzarella, Parmesan, Neufchâtel cheeses) • Regular cottage cheese • Cream, half and half, whipping cream, regular nondairy creamer or flavored creamer, whipped topping, sour cream

Eggs and egg substitutes: no more than two egg yolks per week (four if eggs have added omega-3 fats)	
Foods to eat	*Foods to avoid*
• Egg whites (two whites can substituted for one whole egg in recipes), cholesterol-free egg substitute	• Egg yolks (more than two per week; this includes eggs used in cooking and baking)

Meat and meat substitutes: no more than 6 oz per day	
Foods to eat	*Foods to avoid*
• Lean cuts of well-trimmed beef, pork, lamb (examples: loin or round. Choose select grade, not prime or choice) • Fish or shellfish without butter • Processed meat prepared from lean meats (examples: lean ham, lean hot dogs, lean meat with soy protein added) • Poultry without skin • Tofu, tempeh, vegetable patties • Cooked dried or canned beans (legumes) and peas	• Fatty cuts of beef, pork, and lamb; regular ground beef; spare ribs; organ meats • Fish or shellfish with butter or high-fat sauces

Soups and other mixed dishes: servings per day depend on ingredients	
Foods to eat	*Foods to avoid*
• Reduced-fat or low-fat soups • Soups with less than 600 mg sodium per serving (examples: chicken or beef noodle, minestrone, tomato, vegetable, potato soups)	• Soups made with whole milk, cream, meat fat, poultry fat, or poultry skin • Soups with 600 mg or more sodium per serving

SWEETS AND DESSERTS:
IF YOUR TRIGLYCERIDE LEVELS ARE ABOVE NORMAL, AVOID FOODS IN THIS SECTION. OTHERWISE, EAT ONLY SMALL AMOUNTS.

Foods to eat	Foods to avoid
- Syrup, turbinado sugar, honey, jam, preserves, fruit-flavored gelatin, sucralose (brand name: Splenda), aspartame (brand names: NutraSweet, Equal) - Dark chocolate - Low-fat and nonfat frozen yogurt, low-fat and nonfat ice cream, sherbet, sorbet, fruit ice, frozen ice pops (one brand: Popsicle) - Cookies, cake, pie, and pudding made with egg whites or egg substitute, skim milk or 1 percent milk, and unsaturated oil - Gingersnaps, fig and other fruit bar cookies, fat-free cookies, angel food cake, desserts with no more than 3 grams of fat per serving	- Candy made with milk chocolate, chocolate, coconut oil, palm kernel oil, or palm oil - Milk chocolate - Regular ice cream and frozen treats made with regular ice cream - Commercially baked pies, cakes, doughnuts, high-fat cookies, cream pies - Baked goods made with partially hydrogenated oil.

Reproduced with permission from 'Information from Your Family Doctor: Keeping Your Heart Healthy Through Good Nutrition and Exercise,' January 15, 2006, American Family Physician. Copyright © 2006 American Academy of Family Physicians. All Rights Reserved.

FATS AND OILS:
NO MORE THAN 6 TEASPOONS PER DAY

Foods to eat	*Foods to avoid*
- Unsaturated oils: olive oil, canola oil, peanut oil, soybean oil - Spreads with little or no trans-fatty acids (some brand names: Smart Balance Omega Plus and original, Canola Harvest non-hydrogenated spread, others such as Benecol and Take Control) - Salad dressings made with unsaturated oil, or low-fat or nonfat varieties	- Saturated oils: coconut oil, palm kernel oil, palm oil - Hydrogenated oils - Trans-fatty acids (partially hydrogenated oils) - Butter, lard, shortening, bacon fat, stick margarine, margarine with partially hydrogenated oil - Foods made with olestra (brand name: Olean) should be limited; may cause gastrointestinal symptoms and keep fat-soluble vitamins out of circulation

EXERCISE	
Recommended activities	*Activities to avoid*
- Gardening, cleaning the house, walking, climbing stairs, playing with children, activities with friends and family, raking leaves, walking to the store, parking far away, dancing, shoveling snow, yoga - Cycling, hiking, racquetball, running, swimming, walking, weight training	- Excessive inactivity

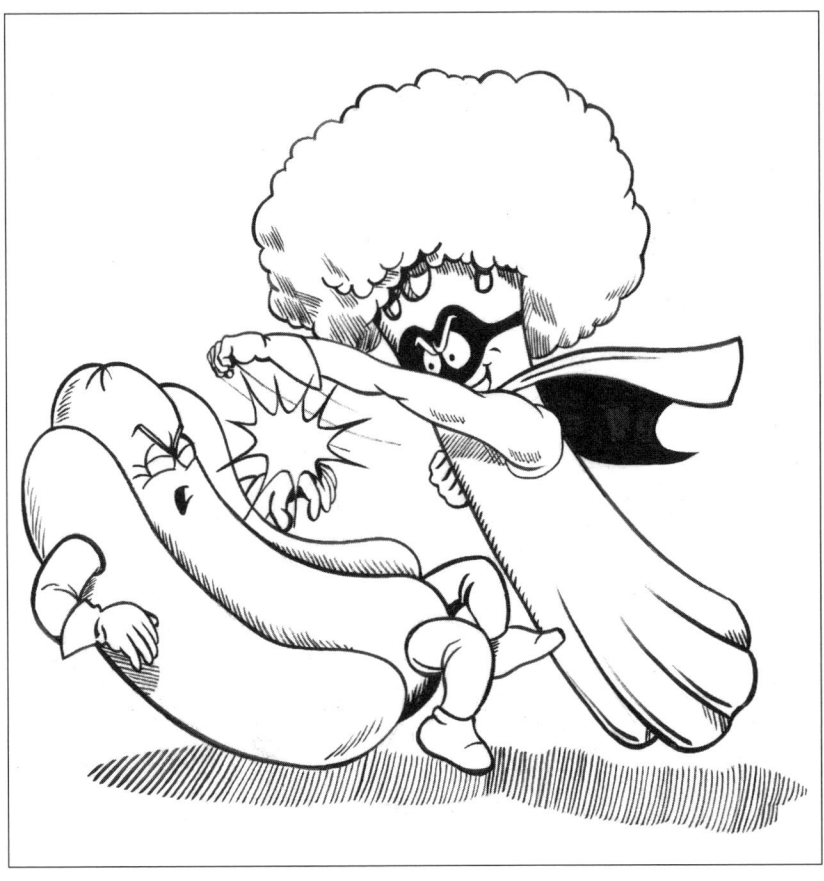

3

Fearless Fiber: Secret Agent

The Diet Fit-Step Mystery Plan has a secret agent called **Fearless Fiber**, who is actually working for our health. This fiber secret agent blocks fat and burns calories for weight-loss, and also contains a multitude of healthy ingredients that prevent many degenerative diseases, including heart disease, high blood pressure, strokes and some forms of cancer. This fiber agent actually helps us to live longer, healthier lives. Fearless Fiber is truly a hero, since it is a secret agent for weight-loss and good health, and is actually more powerful than Agent 007. This secret agent will help your body shed those unwanted pounds quickly and easily.

Fiber is the general term for those parts of plant food that we are unable to digest. Approximately 15% of the starch in foods (known as resistant starch) is tightly bound to fiber and resists the normal digestive processes. Bacteria normally present in the colon ferment this resistant starch and change it into short-chain fatty acids, which are important to normal bowel health and may also help to protect the colon from cancer-causing agents. Foods that contain resistant starch include breads, cereals, pasta, rice, potatoes and legumes. Fiber is not found in foods of animal origin (meats and dairy products). Plant foods contain a mixture of different types of fibers.

These fibers can be divided into soluble or insoluble depending on their solubility in water.

1. **Insoluble fibers:** (cellulose, hemi-celluloses, lignin) make up the structural parts of the cell walls of plants. These fibers absorb many times their own weight in water, creating a soft bulk to the stool and hasten the passage of waste products out of the body. These insoluble fibers promote bowel regularity and aid in the prevention and treatment of some forms of constipation, hemorrhoids, and diverticulitis. These insoluble fibers also may decrease the risk of colon cancer by diluting potentially harmful substances, particularly bile acids, which can cause inflammation and pre-cancerous changes in the lining of the wall of the colon.

2. **Soluble fibers**: (gums, pectins, and mucilages) are found within the plant cells. These fibers form a gel, which slows both stomach emptying and absorption of simple sugars from the intestines. This process helps to regulate blood sugar levels, which is particularly helpful in diabetic patients and is helpful in controlling weight in non-diabetics. Many soluble fibers can also assist in lowering blood cholesterol by binding with bile acids and cholesterol and eliminating the cholesterol through the intestinal tract before the cholesterol can be absorbed into the bloodstream. These soluble fibers actually form a fiber network, like a spider's web, around fatty foods and carry them out of the intestines before they have a chance to be absorbed. Less fat absorbed means lower blood cholesterol and less fat deposited in your body's fat cells. The best sources of soluble fiber are fruits and vegetables, oat bran, barley, dried peas and beans, flax and psyllium seeds.

Two Secret Agents Fight Crime

There are two types of fiber found in all plant foods. Soluble fibers are found in vegetables, all fruits (especially citrus fruits and berries), and flaxseed. Insoluble fibers are found in barley, wheat bran, and other whole grains. Both types of fiber are important in a healthy diet. Your diet should contain at least 35 grams of fiber daily and at least ½ soluble fiber and ½ insoluble fiber. Both types of fiber help to lower fats in the bloodstream, particularly the bad form of cholesterol know as LDL cholesterol. Insoluble fiber helps to transport cholesterol out of the intestinal tract before it can be absorbed into the bloodstream. Soluble fiber helps to break down fats like cholesterol in the intestine so that when they are absorbed they are harmless fats.

New studies have shown that eating more *soluble fiber* found in oranges, apples, figs, and avocados can boost your immune system's cells to fight off bacterial and viral infections. Soluble fiber appears to increase the anti-inflammatory properties of your body's immune cells. Recent research has shown that soluble fiber boosts the body's production of a protein called *interleukin-4*, which stimulates your body's infection-fighting T-cells.

How Fiber Helps You Lose Weight

Weight control is aided by the slower emptying of the stomach when you ingest soluble fibers. This causes a feeling of fullness and a decrease in hunger, causing fewer calories to be consumed. For example, if you eat an apple, which has high fiber content, you'll have a feeling of fullness, as compared to eating a cupcake, which has no fiber, and which is the same weight and size as the apple. In fact, it would take approximately three cupcakes to satisfy your brain's hunger center before you realized that you were full. Well, by then you would already have consumed 480 calories and 17 grams of fat.

A. Fiber helps in weight loss and weight control by the simple fact that high-fiber foods contain **fewer calories for their**

large volume. Fiber-rich foods, such as fruits and vegetables, whole grain cereals and breads, potatoes and legumes are low in fat calories and have high water content. You are, therefore, eating less and enjoying it more.

B. High fiber foods have a **high bulk ratio**, which satisfies the hunger center more quickly than low fiber foods; consequently, fewer calories are consumed. Fiber-rich foods take longer to chew and to digest than fiber-depleted foods, which in turn gives your stomach time to feel full. Feeling full earlier leads to consuming fewer calories. Foods with low-fiber content are, in most cases, considerably more concentrated in calories.

C. The following carbohydrate foods have a **low glycemic index**, and for all intents and purposes can be labeled as good carbs:

- Most vegetables, with the exception of corn and white potatoes.
- Most fruits with the skin intact, with the exception of fruit juices, which contain high levels of sugar and very little actual fruit. Some fruits, for example, watermelon and grapes, do have a high sugar content and have to be consumed in moderation.
- Beans and legumes are excellent sources of fiber, protein, vitamins, minerals, and nutrients.
- Whole grains, including bran, wheat germ, and flax seed.
- Whole-grain cereals, such as oatmeal (instant oatmeals may have a high sugar content) or cold cereals are good choices for low glycemic carbohydrates. Make sure that the package shows a fiber count of at least 5 to 6 grams of fiber, or more, per serving, and a sugar count lower than 10 to 12 grams of sugar per serving, preferably less than 8 grams.
  a. Whole-grain breads. The label on whole-grain breads should show that the first ingredient listed is "whole grain flour." If it doesn't list whole-grain flour first, then it is really not a whole-grain bread. This includes any type of whole-grain bread products.

    b.   Brown long-grain rice makes a good low glycemic addition to any meal, since it is broken down and absorbed slowly.

    c.   Whole wheat pastas now come in many varieties, such as noodles, spaghetti, vermicelli, linguini, etc.

- Nuts are good low glycemic snack foods. In addition to being absorbed slowly, they are excellent sources of protein, fiber, magnesium, copper, folic acid, potassium, and vitamin D. Nuts are also considered to be "the good fats," which are actually called monounsaturated fats. They help to keep the blood vessels open, which, in turn, can reduce the risk of heart disease and strokes. Raw nuts, in particular, are called "heart healthy" nuts, since they contain generous amounts of omega-3 fatty acids. These omega-3 fatty acids are heart protective, and have also been known to prevent certain forms of cancer.

A high-fiber diet is essentially a **healthy, low-fat diet**, which decreases the intake of refined and processed food. This encourages the consumption of fresh fruits, vegetables, and whole-grain cereals and breads. When the fiber is eaten from these food sources, it produces its most beneficial effect, especially when it is eaten with each meal of the day. Dietary fiber takes longer to chew and eat, with the subsequent development of more saliva and a larger bulk swallow with each mouthful. The larger bulk helps to fill the stomach and causes a decrease in hunger before more calories can be consumed. High-fiber diets help to provide bulk without energy and may reduce the amount of energy absorbed from the food that is eaten. These high-fiber diets are often referred to as having a *low-energy density* and appear to prevent excessive caloric (energy) intake. Countries that consume high-fiber diets rarely have obesity problems. The Diet Fit-Step Plan incorporates at least 35 grams or more of fiber into its diet for good health and weight-loss.

Good High-Fiber Carbs

High fiber, good carbs burn more calories during digestion and make you feel fuller earlier and longer than eating refined bad carbs. These good carbs have a *low glycemic index* and are absorbed slowly and cause only a moderate rise in blood sugar and insulin levels. This even level of insulin can **slowly process the blood sugar into the body's cells for energy production** and there is no rapid filling of the cells with fat caused by high levels of sugar and insulin surges, which in turn causes binge carbohydrate eating. Most vegetables (except corn and white potatoes), fruits (not fruit juices), beans, nuts, legumes, chick peas, brown rice, popcorn, whole-grain cereals and breads fall into this category. The good carbs are primarily of plant origin and are naturally low in fat and calories, and contain phyto-nutrients, vitamins, minerals, enzymes and fiber. Many of these good carbohydrates actually contain protein as well.

These good carbs are helpful in a weight-loss program, because your body slowly converts these good carbs into glucose in the intestinal tract, which is then slowly absorbed into the bloodstream. This slow absorption of glucose then causes the pancreas to produce insulin at a steady even level, which results in normal levels of blood sugar and insulin in your bloodstream. Therefore, there is no rapid filling of the fat cells with excess sugar, because there are no spikes in insulin and sugar levels. This results in your appetite being nicely controlled and prevents you from gaining excess weight.

When you consume good carbs (complex carbohydrates) which have a low glycemic index, your body expends 2½ times more energy converting these good carbs from your intestinal tract into energy stores. This means that a high-fiber, complex carbohydrate, low-fat diet causes your body to work that much harder after each meal, burning more calories to produce energy. This in turn boosts your basal metabolic rate which results in the additional burning of about 250 extra calories by the simple thermic action of converting carbohydrates into energy. This means that you are not only consuming less calories by eating good carbs but you are actually burning additional calories just by the simple process of eating and digesting these good carbs. Pretty cool!

Both fiber and protein help to curb your appetite by helping you to feel fuller earlier in the course of your meal. This *fiber-protein combo* slows the rate at which your body absorbs this combination of protein and fiber, thus, minimizing blood sugar and insulin spikes, which can otherwise stimulate your appetite. Also by preventing the production of excess insulin, this fiber-protein combo prevents fat from being deposited in your fat cells, particularly those fat cells located in your abdominal wall. So in effect, you are melting away belly fat as you consume this important fiber-protein combination.

By increasing the lean protein content and decreasing the fat content of your meals, you can slowly and safely lose weight that will stay permanently lost. Unlike low-carb, high-fat diets, you won't experience rapid rebound weight gain that invariably occurs when you stop the diet, and you'll avoid the nasty side effects and hidden health problems inherent in these unsafe low-carb diets. All low-carb diets are high-fat diets and the excess fat calories you eat are stored in your fat cells indefinitely. Complex carbs on the other hand cause your body to work harder during digestion, burning more calories for immediate energy production and for glycogen storage in your muscles and liver for later use.

BAD CARBS & THE GLYCEMIC INDEX

The main element which differentiates bad carbs from good carbs is how fast the carbohydrate foods are converted into sugar in the intestine and absorbed into the bloodstream. This rapid increase in blood sugar causes a rapid increase in insulin levels which in turn causes you to become hungry sooner because of the drop in blood sugar. Excessive calories are then consumed and the excess insulin is produced causing the body fat cells to store more fat, because the production of *glycogen* (stored energy in muscles and liver) is inhibited, which normally causes the body's fat cells to burn stored fuel). Fat cells therefore store more fat instead of burning fat for the production of energy, Result: **Less energy produced, more fat stored**.

The Glycemic Index was developed in order to measure carbohydrate food's effects on blood sugar levels. White flour and white rice, refined highly-processed flour (white breads, cereals, spaghetti, bagels, muffins, pretzels, pancakes), fruit juices and sodas, cakes, pies, ice cream, cookies, candies, chips, and soda have a high-glycemic index, which means that once they pass through the intestinal tract, they are quickly absorbed and cause a rapid spike in blood glucose and insulin levels. Then the rapidly fluctuating glucose and insulin levels lead to excessive calories being consumed, which have no place to go except to be stored in your body's fat cells. This invariably leads to excessive weight gain. High-glycemic diets increase the risk of diabetes, heart disease, strokes and breast cancer. High fiber foods such as whole grain cereals and breads have a low-glycemic index, which causes only a gradual rise in blood sugar and insulin levels. These low-glycemic index foods reduce the risk of developing heart disease and diabetes.

In addition to gaining unwanted pounds, eating foods with a high glycemic index can cause or contribute to health problems. When excess insulin is repeatedly produced by the pancreas by ingesting high-glycemic foods, the pancreas's insulin-producing cells can actually wear out, and then they begin to produce less and less insulin. This can eventually lead to diabetes. Also, overweight and physically inactive people may develop a condition known as *insulin resistance*. This is a condition where the body's tissues resist insulin's signal to transfer glucose from the blood into the cells. This is another way that people on high glycemic diets can develop a condition known as insulin-resistant diabetes. Exercise and weight reduction are certainly ways that this condition can be prevented.

FIBER BLOCK FATS AND BURN CALORIES

Dietary fiber is one of your best foods to block both the absorption of fat and to burn up extra calories. Sounds almost too good to be true; however, it really works. First of all, when you combine the high-fiber foods that we have already discussed (see list of high-fiber foods), combined with any fat in your diet, like a piece of cake or a hamburger, each gram of fiber traps fat globules by entwining them in a fiber-like web, made up of thousands of fiber strands. Once these fat globules are trapped in the fiber's web, they pass through the intestinal tract before they are absorbed into the bloodstream. Therefore, these fat globules are excreted in the waste material from your colon without getting absorbed and stored as fat in your body. The fiber is actually removing the fat from your body like a garbage truck removes garbage. And to underscore that fact, fat really is garbage.

Secondly, fiber actually burns up calories by itself. This is accomplished because fiber causes your intestinal tract to work harder in order to digest the fiber foods. The body's metabolism therefore uses more energy for this time-consuming digestion, and therefore can actually consume most of the calories that the fiber foods contain. Strange as it seems, some heavily fibered foods can actually burn up more calories than the fiber foods contain, thereby creating a deficit of calories. This causes the body to use stored body fat for the production of energy. Each gram of fiber that you consume can burn up approximately 9 calories, most of which come from fat. So if you eat 30 grams of fiber a day, you can actually burn up an additional 270 calories daily (30 grams fiber x 9 calories). You can actually subtract those 270 calories every day from your total daily calorie intake, without actually cutting those calories from your diet. In addition to blocking fat and burning calories, fiber foods bind with water in the intestinal tract and form bulk that makes you feel full early in the course of your meal. So you eat less, and therefore you consume fewer calories at each meal. Also, your appestat (hunger mechanism) is satisfied for longer periods of time, since it takes longer to digest fiber foods, and therefore you will have less of a tendency to snack between meals.

MYSTERY COLORS OF THE SPECTRUM

Many recent medical studies have proved that colorful fruits and vegetables and grains, nuts and seeds, contain disease-fighting substances and can provide a full spectrum of disease prevention. For maximum health benefits, you should eat a variety of vegetables and fruits of many different colors. These colors are formed by pigments in each individual plant. The reason for the different colors is that each colored fruit or vegetable has a different phyto-chemical (phyto means plant). These phyto-chemicals in the fruits and vegetables contain many essential nutrients that help to decrease the risk of heart disease, hypertension, blood clots, degenerative diseases of aging and certain forms of cancer. It is important to eat at least 4-5 servings of fruit or vegetables per day.

The multiple colors of the spectrum found in various fruits and vegetables are derived from their own individual plant pigment. Each one of these colorful fruits and vegetables offer a full spectrum of disease prevention from the phytonutrients and antioxidants found in each plant's beautiful colors. The Diet Fit-Step Plan contains an abundance of all of these healthy nutrients.

The following is a list of some of the phyto-chemicals and antioxidants present in fruits, vegetables, grains and seeds and nuts that can reduce your risk of many diseases:

Spinach If you're looking for a vegetable with super healing powers, try spinach. It's packed with vitamins, antioxidants, and minerals that will protect you from many diseases. Spinach contains many antioxidants including beta and alpha carotenes, lutein, zeaxanthin, potassium, magnesium, vitamin K and folic acid. Recent studies at two major universities have found that, as strange as it seems, spinach may lower the risk of strokes, colon cancer, cataracts, heart disease, osteoporosis, hip fractures, memory loss, Alzheimer's disease, depression and even birth defects. The disease fighting properties in spinach are better absorbed when spinach is cooked with a little olive oil. Now, that's what I call a power vegetable.

Other dark green leafy vegetables (collard greens, kale, bok choy, mustard greens) are low in calories and have high fiber content. These crunchy foods take longer to chew, which helps to shut off the brain's hunger control mechanism (appestat). This fiber also prevents the absorption of fat from the gastro-intestinal tract by wrapping thread like fibers around the fat globules, and quickly eliminates them out of the intestinal tract, before they have a chance to be absorbed.

Kale and **spinach** are two vegetables rich in the antioxidants *lutein* and *zeaxanthin*. These antioxidants have been reported to protect against age-related cataracts and macular degeneration, one of the leading causes of blindness. Also high in these vision-protecting antioxidants are romaine lettuce, broccoli, collards, turnip greens, and corn.

Green leafy vegetables are low in calories and are filling because of their fiber content and their crunch factor. Crunchy fiber foods take longer to eat and help your brain's hunger mechanism to shut down quickly. Fiber also helps to prevent the absorption of fat from the intestinal tract by wrapping threads of fiber around the fat globules, thus preventing the fat's absorption into the blood and actually sweeping the fat through and out of the intestinal tract before it is absorbed. Green leafy vegetables also contain many plant nutrients, antioxidants, and B-complex vitamins, which help to prevent cancer, heart disease, and degenerative neurological diseases.

Broccoli and broccoli sprouts also contain power nutrients that can reduce your risk of heart disease, and certain types of cancer. The active antioxidant in broccoli is *glucoraphanin*, which has been shown to boost your body's defense mechanism against cancer-causing free radicals which damage normal cells in the body. This particular antioxidant also lowers blood pressure, strengthens the immune system, decreases inflammation in the body and has been shown to reduce the incidence of strokes.

Sweet Potatoes: Contrary to popular belief, sweet potatoes are excellent sources of vitamins and minerals and are considered good carbs. They are a great addition to any weight-loss program because of their high fiber content and their nutritional value. Sweet potatoes are good sources of vitamin C, B-complex, folic acid, potassium, vitamin A, and beta-carotene. These nutrients combined with plant sterols, found in sweet potatoes, are powerful antioxidants, which can help to lower cholesterol and lower your risk of heart disease. When sweet potatoes are eaten with their skin, they are good sources of both insoluble and soluble fiber. These two types of fibers help to reduce your appetite the way most fiber foods do, by filling you up and satisfying your appetite early, without supplying extra calories in your diet.

Tomatoes contain the antioxidant *lycopene,* which helps to prevent both prostate and breast cancers. Tomatoes also contain lots of vitamin C, which when combined with lycopene can help to lower your blood cholesterol. Tomatoes are unique in their ability to produce an amino acid called *carnitine.* This amino acid causes your body to burn fat at a faster rate by increasing your body's basal metabolic rate. Any tomato products, from ketchup to tomato sauce, are great for your weight-reducing diet.

Asparagus contains a unique antioxidant called *glutathione,* which helps to fight dangerous free-radicals, which in turn can damage normal cells in your body. Asparagus is a good source of folic acid, potassium, beta-carotene, vitamin C and fiber. Asparagus is a great addition to any diet program, since it is low in calories and high in nutrients. Steamed asparagus is great eaten alone or in a salad. It must be refrigerated or frozen quickly to prevent the loss of its nutritional value. If boiled too long, most of the nutrients end up in the water.

Beans are high in potassium and low in sodium, which helps to reduce your risk of developing high blood pressure and strokes Beans are chock full of fiber which helps to reduce the absorption of fat and unwanted calories from the gastro-intestinal tract. The high fiber content of beans is great for your weight loss plan, since it reduces your appetite by filling you up faster, so that you eat fewer calories. Beans have almost as many calories and as much protein as meat without the added saturated fat. The fiber and water content of beans make you feel fuller earlier in your meal so that you don't consume excess calories. One cup of cooked beans (⅔ of a can) contains 12 grams of fiber whereas meat on the other hand contains no fiber at all. Meat is therefore digested quickly whereas fiber is digested slowly, keeping you satisfied longer. Beans are also low in sugar, which prevents insulin from spiking in the bloodstream and causing hunger pangs.

In a recent study, bean eaters weighed on average, seven pounds less and had slimmer waists than their bean-avoiding counterparts, even though they consumed 200 calories less daily than the non-bean eaters. Beans also contain antioxidants and phytonutrients which fight dangerous free-radicals in your body, which can cause degenerative diseases of aging, cardiovascular diseases, and cancer. The beans which contained the most antioxidants were: red kidney beans, pinto beans, small red beans, navy beans, black beans, and black-eyed peas. Beans have lots of fiber and protein and no fat at all. The perfect combo for a super power food. Beans, beans—they're good for the heart, the more you eat them, the more you're smart!

Peas are packed with vitamins A, B-1, B-6, C, and vitamin K which is known for maintaining strong bones and helping blood to clot in order to prevent bleeding. Peas are high in fiber and are an excellent source of vegetable protein. They also have the added benefit of containing no fat or cholesterol. One cup of peas which contains approximately 100 calories has as much protein as a tablespoon of peanut butter or a ¼ of a cup of nuts. Peas are another example of a super power food even though they're very small. Size doesn't really matter. Other vegetables that are rich sources of Vitamin K are: cabbage, broccoli, spinach, cauliflower, and beans.

Peppers are great sources of vitamins A, C, B-complex, beta-carotene, folic acid and potassium. All colors of sweet peppers (red, yellow, green) are high in fiber and low in calories and are great foods for your Diet Fit-Step weight-loss plan. Peppers contain spices that also can reduce your appetite because they satisfy your taste buds and hunger, before you've had a chance to eat a big meal.

Peppers contain antioxidants that help to prevent blood clots by decreasing the blood platelets' stickiness. This property can help to prevent heart attacks and strokes. Hot peppers contain higher quantities of antioxidants than sweet peppers. They also contain phytonutrients that help to prevent certain forms of cancer. Hot peppers also contain an ingredient called *capsaicin*, which makes these peppers hot and spicy. This ingredient has anti-inflammatory properties and helps to relieve the pain of various forms of arthritis and nerve inflammations. These capsaicinoids can cause eye irritation if transferred from your hands to your eyes, so be careful to wash your hands thoroughly after handling hot peppers.

Soybeans contain soy proteins, which helps to reduce the risk of cardiovascular disease. The reason for this is that soy proteins reduce the amount of total fat and LDL cholesterol in the blood by affecting the synthesis and metabolism of cholesterol in the liver. Its amino acid composition differs from the structure of other proteins found in meat and milk. Clinical trials showed a significantly lower incidence of coronary heart disease in patients with a high soy intake. Soybeans can be found in many different varieties, including soy beverages, tofu, tempeh, soy-based meat substitutes, edamame and hummus. However, to qualify as a heart-healthy food, such soy-rich foods should contain at least 6.5 grams of soy protein, and less than 3 grams of total fat per serving and less than 1 gram of saturated fat per serving. One-half cup of cooked soybeans contains 4 grams of fiber. Soybeans are also a good source of dietary fiber.

In another related study, soy supplements were shown to cut the risk of developing colon cancer in half. Soy supplements also decreased the relative risk of having a recurrence of colon cancer in high-risk subjects. This study was reported at the annual conference of The American Institute for Cancer Research.

Soy contains natural phytonutrients called *isoflavones*. These plant chemicals break down the fat which is stored in your body's fat cells. Several studies have confirmed that the consumption of soy products on a regular basis helps dieters burn fat and lose weight without any other alteration in their diets. These isoflavones present in soy also have been shown to reduce the incidence of heart disease. In addition to helping you lose weight by breaking down the stored fat in your body, isoflavones also break down saturated fat in your blood, thus lowering the LDL bad cholesterol. Soy products (soy milk, soy yogurt, tofu, etc.) are good for heart and great for your figure.

Mushrooms: Many types of mushrooms contain the amino acid *glutamic acid*, which boosts the immune system and helps to fight various types of infections. By helping to improve the body's immune system, mushrooms have also been known to fight certain forms of cancer and autoimmune diseases, such as rheumatoid arthritis, lupus, and other collagen disease. Mushrooms are also rich in potassium and vitamin C, which help to keep blood pressure normal.

Portobello and white mushrooms have a high content of certain nutrients and minerals, particularly *selenium*, which may help to reduce the risk of prostate and breast cancer. When selenium is combined with the vitamin E present in mushrooms, it helps to prevent nasty free radicals from damaging the body's normal cells, thus slowing the aging process. Shiitake mushrooms also contain many plant nutrients, in particular *lentinan* and *eritadenine*, which help to improve the immune system and assist in lowering blood cholesterol. These phytonutrients have also been shown to reduce the risk of heart disease and certain forms of cancer.

All mushrooms are low in calories and are fat-free, making them excellent staples in a weight-loss program. They are excellent flavor enhancers for a variety of foods. Mushrooms are not only good for you, but they are great for your weight-loss program.

Onions and Curry: In a recent study from Johns Hopkins University School of Medicine, it was found that the chemicals found in onions and curry may help to prevent colon polyps. The antioxidant found in onions is called *quercetin*, and the antioxidant found in curry is called *curcumin*. It is thought that these two powerful antioxidants decrease the formation of colon polyps in patients who have an inherited-type of precancerous colon polyps. The average number of polyps decreased by 60% and the average size of the polyps decreased by 50% in patients who consumed these two powerful antioxidants found in both onions and curry.

Grapefruit contains high levels of potassium, vitamin C, beta-carotene, and the antioxidant *lycopene*, which has been shown to reduce the risk of both breast and prostate cancers. Grapefruits also contain bioflavonoids, which appear to protect against heart disease. They also contain phytonutrients, which include *phenolic acid*, which can block nitrosamines, which are cancer-causing chemicals found in many smoked foods.

Grapefruits are a great addition to any weight-reduction program, since they are low in calories and high in fiber. The only precaution is that patients who are on cholesterol-lowering drugs called the statins should be careful about drinking grapefruit juice with these medications. Grapefruit juice appears to slow the natural breakdown of these drugs in the bloodstream, causing higher than expected levels of these medications to stay active in the blood for longer periods of time. It is important for any patient on statin medication to check with their doctor before combining grapefruit with these cholesterol-lowering drugs.

Oranges protect your heart and fight cancer. In a recent study, it was shown that oranges boost HDL cholesterol, in addition to providing vitamin C, folic acid, and numerous flavonoids. These compounds are thought to prevent cholesterol oxidation, which has been linked to a reduced risk of coronary events. An orange or two a day will keep atherosclerosis away. Researchers have found that citrus fruits, in particular oranges, also showed anti-cancer activity in animals and in test tubes. These researchers found that animals that ate oranges for several months were 25% less likely to develop early colon cancer than animals given only water. Compounds such as *liminoids* in oranges seem to alter the characteristics of the colon lining, discouraging cancer growth. These researchers speculate that the orange juice may also help to suppress breast cancer, prostate, and lung cancer.

Blueberries may reverse the aging process. New research has indicated that women on antioxidant-rich diets showed fewer age-related disorders than those on a normal diet. The studies showed that among all the fruits and vegetables, the benefits were greatest with blueberries, which reversed age-related effects; for example, loss of balance and lack of coordination. They also discovered that blueberry extract had the greatest effect on reversing aging decline. Antioxidants help neutralize free radical by-products in the conversion of oxygen into energy, which, if not neutralized, can cause oxidative stress and lead to cell damage. Previous studies have shown that both strawberries and spinach extract can also help to prevent the onset of age-related defects. However, the greatest effect was shown in patients who ate blueberries. Phytonutrients in blueberries, particularly flavonoids and beta-carotene, seem to have an anti-inflammatory effect, which may even help in the prevention of Alzheimer's disease. Again, we have another solid recommendation for eating fruits and vegetables because of their high fiber content and because of their phytonutrients and antioxidants.

Apples: The old adage that, "an apple a day keeps the doctor away," may contain more truth than we actually realize. When you eat an apple with the skin on it every day, you help prevent many health related problems. Apples contain a mysterious antioxidant called *quercetin* which has many beneficial properties. First of all this compound acts as an antihistamine which may help to relieve the symptoms of asthma and other allergy related problems. Quercetin also has anti-inflammatory properties that may reduce the pain associated with arthritis and other inflammatory problems. This unique antioxidant has also been shown to protect the brain cells from circulatory damage, which can help to prevent strokes and reduce the incidence of age-related neurological disorders such as Alzheimer's disease. And finally, quercetin has been shown to prevent certain forms of cancer, including breast and prostate cancer.

Apples, because of their high water and fiber content, will help you to lose weight and also help to lower your blood pressure. Apples also help to fight inflammation in the muscles of the body which can cause an increase in the enzyme CRP (C-reactive protein). This enzyme can be responsible for heart attacks and even some forms of arthritis like rheumatoid arthritis.

Fruits and vegetables in general contain various healthy antioxidants and phytonutrients that prevent many cardiovascular and degenerative diseases of aging, including several forms of cancer.

New studies have also shown that fruits can prevent or reduce the incidence of uterine fibroids, which are the most commonly diagnosed uterine tumors. These tumors have been associated with anemia, pelvic pain, and in some cases, fertility problems. It appears that women who have high levels of estrogens, which may be related to high meat intake, are more prone to fibroids. A recent study showed that diets decreasing or eliminating meats and increasing green vegetables have a significant effect on the prevention of the development of fibroids. The vegetables and fruits contain *isoflavinoids*, which can offset the effect of estrogen on the body. Also, by eliminating meat from the diet, the levels of estrogen in the body decrease. By decreasing meat and increasing fiber, the body is less likely to develop estrogen-related uterine fibroid tumors.

Veggies and fruits also help prevent breast and uterine cancer. Women who limit their intake of red meat and eat lots of green vegetables have a reduced risk of developing breast cancer and uterine cancer. High levels of estrogen, which results from the consumption of beef, ham, pork, and other red meat, have been implicated in the formation of breast and uterine cancer. The intake of 4-5 servings of fruits and vegetables daily with phytonutrients, in particular, isoflavinoids, may offset some of estrogen's effect on the uterus and breast.

Cruciferous vegetables also decrease the risk of bladder cancer. In a recent study on bladder cancer, it was shown that in order to reduce the risk of bladder cancer, it is necessary to drink lots of fluids, not to smoke, and to eat lots of cruciferous vegetables. A high intake of cruciferous vegetables, particularly **broccoli** and **cabbage**, significantly reduced the risk of bladder cancer. This may be explained by the presence of one or more phytochemicals in broccoli and cabbage, which are specific in the reduction of bladder cancer risk. This study also showed that a high intake of fruits, yellow vegetables, and green, leafy vegetables did not significantly reduce the risk of bladder cancer. The relationship with high cruciferous vegetable intake (broccoli and cabbage) was associated with the highest reduction in the risk of developing bladder cancer.

In a recent study reported in the Journal of the American

Medical Association, it appears that people, who eat foods that are high in *plant based estrogen*, appear to have a lower incidence of lung cancer. Broccoli, cabbage, soy products, spinach and chick peas are excellent sources of plant based estrogens. Vegetables in general are low in calories and high in fiber, making them excellent choices for a healthy weight-loss program.

Nuts have a low glycemic index and are absorbed slowly. They are also a good source of protein and contain many essential nutrients such as fiber, copper, magnesium, folic acid, vitamin D and E, and potassium. Nuts, particularly walnuts and almonds, contain heart-healthy monounsaturated fats. These good fats can lower blood cholesterol, prevent heart disease and reduce the incidence of high blood pressure. Nuts actually help to retain the natural elasticity of the blood vessels which helps to lower the blood pressure. Nuts, especially walnuts have a high content of an amino acid called *L-argentine* and also contain *alpha-linolenic* acid, which is a plant-based omega-3 fatty acid. These two compounds help to dilate your arteries and offer additional heart-protective properties as well as to help prevent certain forms of cancer.

Nuts are also an excellent source of protein, which act as a natural appetite suppressant, because of its slow digestion and absorption into the bloodstream. Most of the energy contained in the protein in nuts is burned as fuel for all of your body's metabolic functions. Therefore, hardly any of the calories contained in the dietary protein found in nuts is converted into fat storage, which is why nuts are a good addition to the Diet Fit-Step weight-loss plan.

Frequent consumption of walnuts (four to five servings per week) has been shown to reduce the risk of coronary heart disease by as much as 50%. Nuts also have been shown to decrease both the total cholesterol by 5-10% and the LDL cholesterol by 15-20%. A study published in *The Journal of Nutrition* indicated that of all edible plants, walnuts have one of the highest concentrations of antioxidants. In a more recent study reported in the *Journal of Circulation*, from the Hospital Clinic of Barcelona, Spain, Dr. Emilio Ros said that, "This is the first time a whole food, not its isolated components, has shown this beneficial effect on vascular health." He further stated that, "Walnuts differ from all other nuts because of their high content of alpha-linolenic acid (ALA), a plant-based omega-3 fatty acid, which may provide additional heart-protective properties." Several other beneficial components of walnuts include: L-arginine, which may be cardio protective by dilating the arteries. Walnuts also contain fiber, folic acid, gamma-tocopherol, and other antioxidants, which also help to prevent atherosclerosis (hardening of the arteries).

Sunflower Power: Sunflower seeds contain many healthy nutrients including the healthy monounsaturated fatty acids. These seeds are excellent sources of the B vitamins: thiamine, folate, and pantothenic acids, and the minerals copper, zinc, iron, and selenium.

One ounce of sunflower seeds daily provides all of these essential vitamins and minerals in addition to the heart-protective antioxidant vitamin E. Sunflower seeds and oil contain both mono and polyunsaturated fats which can reduce LDL (bad cholesterol) and increase beneficial HDL (good cholesterol) in the blood.

Whole grains: In a recent study in the American Journal of Clinical Nutrition, women who ate three to four servings of whole grains a day had one-third to one-half the risk of developing heart disease as opposed to women who ate refined flour, such as white bread. It is important to check the ingredients in any commercial food to see that it is truly made from whole grains. In particular, it is important to check the ingredients in snack foods (for example, cookies, crackers, and chips), since many of these products contain not only refined white flour, but also partially hydrogenated oils (trans-fats), which actually can raise our cholesterol more than other types of saturated fats.

Recent studies have subsequently shown that high fiber diets, which include not only cereal grains, but fruits and vegetables, do, indeed, help to prevent against the development of colon cancer. As part of the ongoing Nurses' Health Study that provided the data questioning the preventive role of fiber, a recent report showed that women who ate a diet high in red meat had higher rates of colorectal cancer. In that same study, women whose diets were low in red meat and high in fruits, vegetables, and cereal grains had a significantly decreased risk of colon cancer. In countries where diets are high in plant-based foods and low in red meat and animal fat, people have lower rates of heart disease and colon cancer.

Oatmeal has a high content of insoluble fiber which makes it an excellent food for your Diet Fit-Step Plan. Oatmeal has a high content of insoluble fiber, which helps to shut off your appetite control mechanism because oatmeal is absorbed slowly from the intestinal tract. Oatmeal also has a high soluble fiber content, which helps to increase the good (HDL) cholesterol which in turn flushes out the bad (LDL) cholesterol from your bloodstream. Oatmeal and other high fiber, bran cereals are also loaded with the mineral magnesium, which helps to regulate your insulin levels and reduces your risk of developing diabetes and obesity. Oatmeal is also high in soluble fiber, which helps to clean out the fat in your blood vessels by increasing the HDL cholesterol, which sweeps out the bad LDL cholesterol from the bloodstream.

Oatmeal for breakfast every day has been recommended by the American Heart Association as a great start for your day to reduce your risk of heart disease. People who eat oatmeal, as well as other whole-grain bran-type cereals daily, have less than one-half the risk of developing obesity and diabetes as non-cereal eaters. High-fiber bran cereals help to regulate insulin production in the morning. This helps to control your appetite and reduce the risk of gaining unwanted pounds. Bran cereals are also packed with magnesium, which is a mineral that can also reduce your risk of developing diabetes. Magnesium also helps to stabilize your blood sugar by preventing the overproduction of insulin by the pancreas. Oatmeal and whole-grain bran-type cereals are a great way to start your diet every morning. Fiber-rich oatmeal is nutritious, tastes great, and is slow to digest. The high insoluble fiber content of oatmeal causes your appetite mechanism to shut down early because of its slow rate of absorption from the intestinal tract. Oatmeal has also been shown to reduce your craving for high-refined sugar products and fatty foods.

HEALTHY ANTIOXIDANT SECRET FOODS

FRUITS	VEGGIES	OTHERS
Apples	Avocados	Canola oil
Apricots	Beans	Dates & figs
Blackberries	Bok Choy	Flax seeds
Blueberries	Broccoli	Garlic
Cantaloupe	Cabbage	Ginger
Cherries	Carrots	Nuts
Cranberries	Cauliflower	Olive oil
Mangoes	Greens (others)	Peanut oil
Oranges	Kale	Raisins
Prunes	Spinach	Soy beans
Purple grapes	Squash	Tea
Raspberries	Sweet potatoes	Whole grains
Strawberries	Tomatoes	

THE MYSTERY DIETS OF TWO COUNTRIES

THE MEDITERRANEAN DIET

Research shows that the Mediterranean diet, which emphasizes whole grains, greens, fruits, vegetables, fish and olive oil, is healthier than the typical American diet, which is high in fat and processed foods. There is a significantly decreased risk of heart disease and cancer in the Mediterranean cultures, which have been thriving on these foods for thousands of years. The Mediterranean diet has been found to help protect against heart disease and helps to control blood cholesterol and blood sugar levels. In the Mediterranean diet, people consume at least 25-30 grams of fiber a day. In addition to fiber, this diet is rich in **omega-3 fatty acids** from fish oils and **alpha-linoleic acid** from plant sources. Both of these substances help fiber to reduce the incidence of heart disease. The Mediterranean diet is far superior to our western diet, and shows us why fiber is a significantly important factor in the Diet Fit-Step Plan.

The Mediterranean diet is rich in **olive oil**, which is a heart-healthy monounsaturated fat that helps to increase your body's good cholesterol (HDL) and decrease the bad cholesterol (LDL). This decreases your risk of heart attacks and strokes by decreasing cholesterol deposits in your arteries. The Mediterranean people use olive oil on almost everything they eat (pastas, breads, salads, vegetables, fish) and even pastries are made with olive oil. They also use olives abundantly in their salads and with their main courses. These people also eat considerable less saturated fat than most countries, including the United States. And the Mediterranean people have one more secret besides their diet that keeps them healthy and free of many of the diseases of aging. It's **walking**, of course. Mediterranean people, in addition to eating healthy, walk all of the time. They walk to work, to visit friends, to shop or just to take a carefree walk. Walking is just a natural part of their lives. They frequently walk hills, because of the Mediterranean terrain.

In a recent edition of the *Journal American Medical Association*, it was reported that elderly people who followed the Mediterranean diet (olive oil, nuts, seeds, whole grains, vegetables, greens, fish and fruit) and walked 30-40 minutes every day, had a 65% lower mortality rate than a similar age group of people who ate a typical American high fat, low fiber diet and were also sedentary. These individuals who followed the Mediterranean diet had a significant decrease in body weight, blood cholesterol and triglycerides, blood pressure, blood sugar and insulin levels. They also had a significant increase in their good cholesterol (HDL) and a decrease in their bad cholesterol (LDL), both of which help to decrease the risk of heart disease and strokes. This particular study followed over 2,500 men and women, ages 70-90, in 11 different European countries for a period of 12 years.

In a similar study also reported in the *Journal American Medical Association*, it was found that people on the Mediterranean diet reduced their risk of developing the **metabolic syndrome.** This condition occurs when excess amounts of fat accumulate around the abdomen because of the body's resistance to insulin due to a high fat, low fiber diet. This syndrome increases a person's risk for developing hypertension, coronary heart disease, diabetes, obesity certain forms of cancer and dementia. In two separate studies reported in the *Journal of the American Medical Association*, it was reported that the mortality rates were 65% lower among elderly people who followed the Mediterranean diet combined with 30 minutes of daily exercise, moderate alcohol consumption and no smoking. This diet consists primarily of olive oil rather than butter or margarine, legumes, nuts, seeds, grains, fish, vegetables and potatoes.

THE FRENCH PARADOX

People who ate a diet that was rich in purple grapes had an almost tripling of the blood vessels' ability to respond to an increased blood flow, and also showed a slower onset of LDL oxidation, meaning that it is less likely that the oxidation will contribute to atherosclerosis. The flavinoid *(resveratrol)* in purple grapes is the key to the prevention of atherosclerosis. Fruits, vegetables, nuts, and seeds also contain similar flavinoids, as well as red wine. This research is often referred to as the French Paradox, which helps to explain the low incidence of heart disease in France, where red wine consumption is high. While people in France eat almost 1½ times as much saturated fat as Americans, the French have only ⅓ the risk of heart disease. The same heart disease prevention benefits appear to be related to the consumption of purple grapes, which contain the same resveratrol ingredient as red wine. Eating red grapes or grape juice gives the same protection against heart disease as drinking wine, without the alcohol content.

In addition to drinking red wine, the French people eat a healthy high fiber diet, with lots of vegetables, and fruits. They also add heart-healthy olive oil, nuts, seeds, herbs and spices to their foods. The French usually sauté or grill their vegetables, fish and meat to bring out the natural flavors of the food. They rarely eat pre-packaged processed foods, which are extremely high in saturated fats. Even though the French people like to add sauces to their food, they eat relatively small portions of fatty meats in comparison to the amount of vegetables that they consume. They also take considerable time in preparing and enjoying their meals as compared to the American people, who are always in a hurry to eat their meals and then run off to do something else. It may in fact be, that the French people's relaxed style of eating contributes to their lower incidence of heart disease as compared to the American people with their frenetic lifestyles.

FIBER DECREASES ALL CAUSES OF MORTALITY

In a recent study in the American *Journal of Epidemiology*, individuals on a high fiber diet showed a significantly reduced risk from coronary heart disease and death from all causes. This study reviewed dietary data from the Scottish Heart Study on approximately 12,000 women and men ages 40 to 59 years of age. These results suggest that the current public health drive to increase your fiber intake to at least five portions of fruits and vegetables a day should have beneficial effects on all causes of mortality.

These researchers attributed the beneficial effects of fiber to the fact that folate, the antioxidant active flavinoids, and minerals (selenium, magnesium and copper) will be co-ingested at higher levels in high-fiber, fruit and vegetable-rich diets. In addition, the stool-bulking properties of fiber may play an important role. Along with fiber, the study participants ingested other nutrients present in fruits and vegetables that may have an added effect on the prevention of coronary heart disease and on all types of mortality. The antioxidant vitamin E showed the strongest beneficial effect with vitamin-C and beta-carotene. This study also showed that consuming high levels of fiber and antioxidants were associated with significantly lower rates of coronary heart disease and all types of mortality.

CRP or C-reactive protein is a measure of inflammation that occurs in your body if you have heart disease, high blood pressure, diabetes, or obesity. Adults with these medical conditions, who had a low fiber intake, are two to three times as likely to have an elevated CRP level compared with people who had none of these conditions. There is considerable medical evidence that dietary fiber reduces both inflammation in the body and also reduces blood cholesterol levels. The American Heart Association and the American Diabetes Association both recommend that adults should consume at least 30 to 35 grams of fiber per day. So in addition to its long line of health benefits (lower blood pressure, low heart disease risk, low cholesterol levels, improved GI function, weight control, etc.), fiber now has the unique distinction of lowering the levels of a very dangerous component in the blood, namely c-reactive protein. CRP also may actually be implicated in contributing to other degenerative diseases of aging including arthritis and cancer.

The nutrients in fruits and vegetables, such as dietary fiber and antioxidants, are associated with a lower risk of heart disease, but few studies have examined their relationship to the risk for stroke. This study, reported in the *Journal of the American Medical Association*, described the association between fruit and vegetable intake and ischemic stroke in over 75,000 woman enrolled in the Nurses' Health Study and 38,000 men in the health professional follow-up study. Everyone in this particular study had no history of cardiovascular disease, stroke, cancer, diabetes, or high cholesterol. During the follow-up period, which included fourteen years for women and eight years for men, each increment of one serving of fruit or vegetables per day was associated with a 7% reduction for risk of ischemic stroke in women, and a 4% reduction in men. This would translate into a *35% reduction in stroke for women* who ate five servings daily of fruit and vegetables. This study showed that there was no further reduction in the risk of stroke above 5-6 servings of fruit and vegetables per day. The consumption of a variety of vegetables and fruits, such as cruciferous vegetables (examples: broccoli and cabbage), green, leafy vegetables, citrus fruits or vitamin C-rich fruits and vegetables resulted in the largest decrease in risk. Pretty impressive results for sticking to your high-fiber diet of fruits and veggies.

ADD LOTS OF FIBER TO YOUR DIET

1. **Drink 6-8 glasses of water daily.** Fiber can absorb many times its own weight of water, providing bulk to the diet and a subsequent feeling of fullness. A high fiber diet requires that you drink lots of water, so that the fiber can absorb much of the water and create bulk in the intestines, which makes you feel full, before you've had a chance to eat too much. Although drinking a lot of water (six 8 ounce glasses per day) will quench your thirst, it will not satisfy your hunger; however, if you eat foods with high water content, you will feel full earlier and subsequently eat less food. It's the combination of the water in the fruits and vegetables that satisfies your hunger mechanism. So, in effect, you're eating foods with extra volume without extra calories. If you fill up with foods that have high water content, you'll take in fewer calories without feeling hungry. You can actually eat more foods than you're eating now, that will make your hunger go away while you still lose weight in the process. The key factor is to eat foods that contain a lot of water, such as vegetables and fruits

2. **Eat high-fiber whole grain cereals for breakfast**, preferably those with 5 or more grams of fiber per serving. Be careful of so-called, "healthy granola cereals," many of which have a high saturated fat content and little fiber. Some granola cereals; however, are low in fat and high in fiber. Always check the ingredients label. *Cereals with 5 or more grams fiber:* shredded wheat, puffed wheat, steel-cut oats, All Bran®, Fiber One®, Raisin Bran®, All Bran®, Multi-Grain Wheat Check®, Multi-Grain Cheerios®, Bran Flakes®, Kashi® and soy, fax seed and whole grain bran cereals.

3. **Breads must have the word "whole"** listed as the first ingredient on the package; otherwise it's not a true whole-grain product, no matter how the bread is labeled. Substitute whole grain bread (stone ground or whole wheat) or fiber enriched bread and bran instead of white refined breads.

Always use whole grain or fiber-enriched breads, which have more than double the fiber content of white bread. *Use whole grain flour or soy flour* instead of refined white flour. Eat whole grain pastas in place of regular pasta. Use whole grain products (bran and whole grain cereals, brown long grain rice, and whole grain noodles).

4. **Eat fresh fruit with skin**, rather than fruit juices, which have little or no fiber content. Increase fruits (apples, oranges, pears, bananas, strawberries, blueberries, plums, peaches, plums, prunes, and cherries). Fruits with a high volume of water include watermelons, strawberries, blueberries, blackberries, peaches, oranges, cantaloupe, apples, grapes, bananas and pears. Vegetables with a high content of water include squash, carrots, broccoli, asparagus, sweet potatoes, beans, corn on the cob, avocados and peas. Many fad diets restrict fruits because they contain sugar; however, fruits have natural sugars like fructose, which are not that high in calories. Fruits also contain a high content of water and fiber which fills you up quickly and satisfies your hunger mechanism before you've eaten too many calories. Also, fruits contain antioxidants, vitamins and other essential nutrients for good health.

5. **Consume more vegetables**, legumes and salads (without the dressing, of course, unless you use a little olive oil and vinegar). Include carrots, celery, cabbage, peas, broccoli, Brussels sprouts, lentils, potatoes with skin, dried beans and baked beans (without sugar or bacon). Add other garden vegetables such as green beans, lettuce, onions, corn, peas, tomatoes, and spinach.

6. Add bran, wheat germ, nuts, seeds, legumes, beans or grits to soups (not creamed), yogurt or casseroles. **Unprocessed bran and wheat germ** are dry bran/wheat powders, which are convenient, high dietary fibers. and contain approximately 2 grams of dietary fiber per tsp. Either may be sprinkled on any cereal or other foods, or may be mixed in with orange or tomato juice to improve its taste.

7. **Snack foods** with a high fiber count include dried fruits, nuts, seeds, bran cereals, cereal-fruit-bars (high-fiber, low-fat), rice cakes, celery, carrot sticks and popcorn. *Popcorn* is an excellent high-fiber, low-fat, low-calorie snack. Use non- or low-fat varieties. Without the added salt, oil, and butter, popcorn is probably one of the best diet snacks available. It is low in calories and cholesterol, and high in fiber. It consequently fills you up without adding extra calories and provides 2 grams of fiber per 1½ cups. One cup of popcorn contains only 25 calories. The electric hot-air popper is, by far, the most efficient way to prepare popcorn. Since it uses no oil or butter, there are no added fats, and there is no cleanup necessary. These hot-air poppers can produce great quantities of popcorn in a relatively short period of time. Many microwaveable popcorn varieties contain considerable fat; however, several newer products are available in low-fat varieties. Always check the label.

8. Start **adding fiber slowly** to your diet to avoid cramping, bloating, or gas. Make small additions of fiber-rich foods over a period of four to six weeks. If you find that a particular high-fiber food causes cramping or bloating, discontinue eating it and try another type of high-fiber food. Continue to increase your daily fiber intake until you reach 35 grams of fiber a day for good health and weight reduction. Remember, it's very important to drink more fluids as you increase your fiber intake. This excess bulk formed by fiber and water also helps to keep your intestinal tract healthy. The Diet Fit-Step Plan adds the necessary fiber in your diet, which helps you lose weight, stay healthy, live longer, and get rid of those unwanted pounds permanently.

78 THE CASE OF THE UNWANTED POUNDS

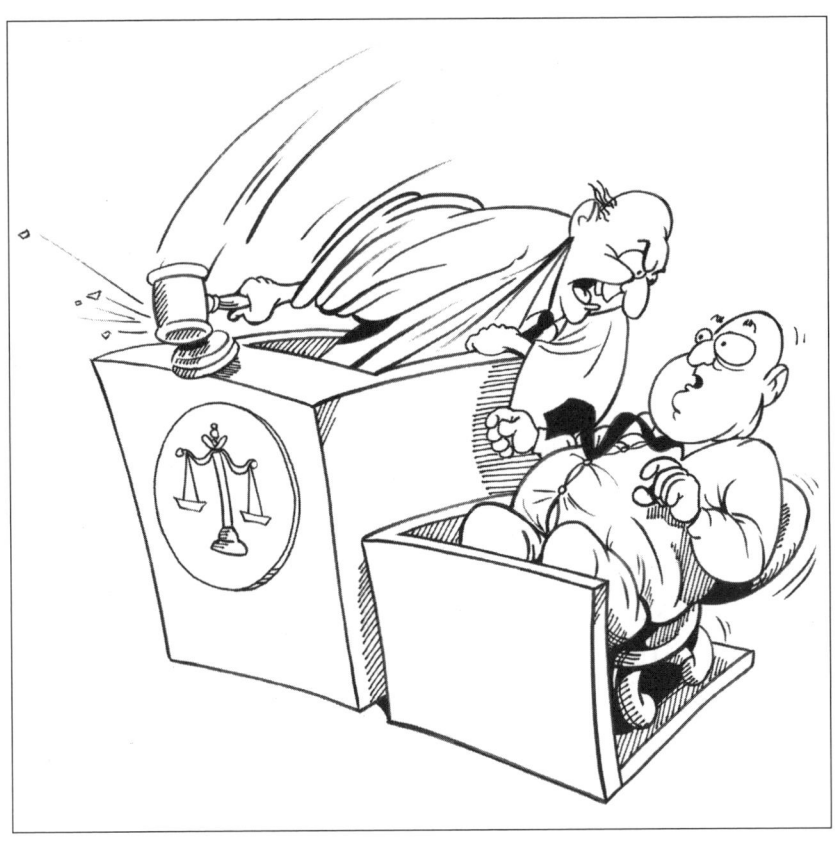

"You're guilty of murder!"

4

Mr. Fat: Guilty of Murder!

Mr. Fat is actually guilty of murder. Your own murder in fact. Dietary fat contributes to the following deadly consequences: obesity, hypertension, strokes, coronary heart disease, heart failure, diabetes, the metabolic syndrome, neurological diseases of aging like Alzheimer's disease, and certain forms of cancer. Remember, the fat you eat will not only make you gain weight, it also puts your health at considerable risk.

In a study just released by the National Heart, Lung and Blood Institute in Bethesda, Maryland, obesity has now been listed as a major independent risk factor for heart disease. What's so new about that? Everyone knows that being overweight contributes to heart disease. That's just it; up until now obesity was just a contributing factor in heart disease because of its relationship with high blood pressure and high cholesterol. Now it has gained its own independent rating as causing heart disease all by itself. This study, consisting of 5,000 women and men, was followed for 26 years. The risk of developing heart disease was more pronounced in people who gained most of their excess weight after the age of 25. In this study, obesity ranked third in men and fourth in women in predicting coronary heart disease. The other factors in heart disease were high blood pressure, serum cholesterol, cigarette smoking, age, diabetes and electrocardiogram abnormalities. Only high blood pressure, cholesterol and age were ranked ahead of obesity with cigarette smoking a close fourth in predicting heart disease. One important point made in this extensive study was: losing a moderate amount of weight lessened the risk of developing heart disease.

According to the American Heart Association, more than 41 million Americans have one or more forms of heart or blood vessel disease. **Heart attacks** claimed 650,000 lives in 2008, 56 percent of all deaths from cardiovascular disease. The Heart Association estimated that as many as one million Americans will have a heart attack this year and more than one-third of them will die.

Stroke was listed as the second leading cause of death in cardiovascular disease, which claimed 195,000 lives in 2008. They estimated that 1.8 million Americans are survivors of stroke. **High Blood Pressure**: one in every four adults or 35 million Americans suffer from high blood pressure. In 2008, over 275,000 people died from the complications of high blood pressure.

Mr. Fat's Accomplice Cholesterol

1. The Framingham Heart Study, which has been in progress for the past 25 years and has followed over 5,000 people, has repeatedly shown that the blood cholesterol level is one of the strongest predictors of a person's risk for developing coronary heart disease. In this study, cholesterol is coupled with other risk factors such as blood pressure, smoking, family history, and lack of exercise.

2. In people who have heart disease at very young ages or in families where there is a high prevalence of heart disease, cholesterol levels are usually found to be high. Epidemiological studies comparing different nations and cultures show that populations who have a high fat intake have significantly more heart disease than cultures with less fat in their diets. In addition, when certain ethnic groups migrate to a new cultural society, they tend to develop both the cholesterol blood levels and risks of heart disease of their new environments.

This suggests that environmental factors such as high cholesterol diets may be more crucial than genetic factors in determining the risk of developing heart disease.

3. There appears to be little doubt from this evidence that the relationship of high levels of blood cholesterol to the development of coronary heart disease is a significant risk factor. The major factor in reducing the level of cholesterol in the blood is to reduce the amount of total fat in the diet and increase the total amount of fiber in the diet by following the **Diet-Step: 35 Grams Fat/35 Grams Fiber Diet.** This usually means consuming less animal fats and whole milk dairy products, and eating more fruits, vegetables, and whole grain products.

4. A second important factor in determining the level of blood cholesterol is the type of fat eaten. Most animal fats are saturated fats, whereas most vegetable oils are monounsaturated or polyunsaturated fats. Studies have shown that substituting monounsaturated fats and to a lesser extent polyunsaturated fats for saturated fats, results in lowering the blood cholesterol level, even if the total amount of fat in the diet is the same. Monounsaturated heart-healthy fats may play an even more important role in the prevention of heart disease, by raising the good HDL cholesterol. And last but not least, is your 35 minute **Fit-Step walking program,** six days per week. Walking not only provides cardiovascular fitness, but it also raises the HDL (good cholesterol-submarine) level in our blood. HDL seems to protect our coronary arteries from accumulating too much cholesterol. Walking also significantly decreases the LDL bad cholesterol.

Mr. Fat's Hide-Out

When you eat a lot of fatty foods, the fat accumulated has to go someplace. You can see what's happening on the outside of your body, now let's take a look at the inside. Fat infiltrates the liver and other organs. It's a squeeze process, an invasion. Fat compresses the heart and lungs, and decreases the blood supply to the rest of the body. Some very obese people can't sit, because if they do, there's no space for their lungs to expand, as the fat invades the chest. These people have to stand up or lie down all the time. They have disabled themselves. Along with all this, extra heavy people, and even moderately overweight persons, are putting an extra burden on their backs and legs (the weight bearing joints), which causes or increases arthritic problems. Complications following surgery occur more frequently in obese people. Wounds don't heal as well or as fast. And again, if there is a breathing problem; overweight people can't take anesthesia as well as people of normal weight.

At a recent American Heart Association meeting, a study showed that men and women store fat in different places: men are more likely to store fat in their abdomens, whereas women store fat more easily in their buttocks and thighs, because nature gave women more fat cells there. What's the significance of these findings? Extra abdominal fat increases the risk of stroke, high blood pressure, diabetes and high cholesterol levels. The extra fat stored by women in the thighs and buttocks appear to be a harmless place to store fat according to this study; however, no woman wants to have fat thighs and buttocks. The good news is that women who walk seem to lose weight more easily in those trouble spots, the thighs and buttocks, making these areas firm and trim. So no matter whether the fat's in your belly or in your buttocks, walking keeps you slim and trim.

FAT MAKES YOU FAT!

The typical American diet has a higher fat content than in nearly any other country in the world. There is little doubt that this increased fat intake in our diet is responsible for the development of obesity, as well as many other disorders. It is important to note that fat is the most concentrated source of calories, since a gram of dietary fat supplies your body with **9 calories**. This is compared to only 4 calories contained in each gram of protein or carbohydrate. Since fat has this concentrated source of calories, it is the most fattening type of food that we can consume, and it stands to reason that cutting down on the total fat intake is one of the best ways to cut down on the total amount of calories, and to lose and maintain normal body weight.

It's very difficult to imagine how many fat calories that you consume each day. It's important to be able to find the fat in your diet and eliminate it. Everyone knows that there's fat in meat, sausage, bacon, lunchmeats, eggs, butter, ice cream, milk and cheese. But not everyone realizes that there's considerable fat in donuts, cakes, pies, muffins, margarine, mayonnaise, chicken and tuna salad, coffee creamers, yogurt, cream cheese and cottage cheese. The more fat calories you consume, the more fat will be stored in your body, and the more weight you will gain. Dietary fat just fills up your fat cells because hardly any of the fat calories (only five out of 1,000) are used for digestion and are therefore not burned up. In other words dietary fat not only is unhealthy, but it actually makes you fat.

Controlling our weight by reducing the amount of saturated fat in our diet has a two-fold benefit. First of all, it will help to control and maintain our weight. Secondly, it will have the beneficial effect of the prevention of cardiovascular and cerebrovascular disease (heart attacks and strokes), since these illnesses have been associated with high levels of blood cholesterol, which, in turn, come from the consumption of saturated fats. In general, we burn almost all of the protein and carbohydrates that we eat every day. We store the remaining carbohydrates in our muscles and liver in the form of a chemical compound called glycogen. This glycogen is used for the future production of energy. The difference between the energy supplied by protein and carbohydrates in our diets, and our total energy needs each day has to come from burning fats.

Weight gain actually occurs from taking in more calories in the form of dietary fats than were burned off as fuel for energy. On a low-fat diet, calories are removed from storage in fat cells and are added to the fuel mixture of protein and carbohydrate for the production of energy. This results in permanent weight loss, unlike the temporary water weight loss of low-carbohydrate diets. Therefore, the less fat that you eat, results in more storage fat being burned as fuel, and subsequently less fat is stored in your body. On the other hand, the more fat that you eat results in more fat being stored and less fat being burned, and consequently more fat cells remain in the form of fatty deposits throughout your body.

Whereas almost none of the calories contained in protein in our diets are converted into storage fat cells, almost 95% of the dietary fat can be stored in fat cells when you take in excess calories of fat in your diet. In other words—**it is the fat in your diet that makes you fat.** It is not necessarily the actual number of calories in your diet that makes you fat, it is the number of fat calories that makes you fat. Fat is stored in fat cells called adipose tissue, in a ratio of four parts fat and one part water. *Since there are 9 calories in each gram of fat,* it means that one pound of fat contains 3,500 calories. It therefore takes a deficit, or reduction, of 3,500 calories to lose this one pound of fat. The only way to lose even one pound of body weight is to burn approximately 3,500 calories. This can only be accomplished by cutting back on the total amount of fat in the diet, and also by increasing your physical activity. Nothing else works!

One of my favorite sayings to my patients when they ask me how to lose weight is: "The only way you can lose weight safely is to eat less fat and to walk more, or, if you would like, you can walk more and eat less fat!" There is little doubt that a **low-fat, high-fiber, and lean-protein diet** is the healthiest, safest, and most effective weight reduction program. This plan is designed for quick weight-loss without rebound weight gain. The Diet Fit-Step Plan consists of eating no more than 35 Grams of Fat and no less than 35 Grams Fiber. When this diet is combined with walking for 35 minutes, 6 days per week and also walking with hand-held weights, 2 or 3 days per week (chapter 10), you have the perfect combination of a double blast of calorie burning. First you burn calories by the actual aerobic exercise of walking. Secondly, you burn additional calories by building muscle tissue with the strength training exercise of walking with weights. You can actually *lose up to 15 pounds and 3 inches in only 21 days* on the Diet Fit-Step Mystery Plan and keep off those unsightly unwanted pounds permanently.

TYPES OF FATS

I. SATURATED FAT

Saturated fat is present in all products of animal origin: meat, fish, fowl, eggs, butter, milk, cream and cheese. Saturated fats are also found in some vegetable products, which are usually solid or semi-solid at room temperature. They include shortenings and table spreads which have been changed from liquid fats (usually cottonseed and soybean oils) into solids by a process called hydrogenation. This process makes the products more suitable for table use and prevents them from becoming rancid. However, this process converts polyunsaturated fats into saturated fats. Other saturated fats in the vegetable kingdom include cocoa butter, palm oil and coconut oil. Most people are unaware of the fact that they consume significant amounts of coconut and palm oil. It is used commercially in a wide variety of processed foods, baked goods and deep-fat fried products.

Saturated fats are dangerous because they can increase the amount of cholesterol in the blood. These fats can raise the level of blood cholesterol as much as, if not more than, the actual consumption of dietary cholesterol products. These fats can also interfere with brain function and can actually cause damage to the brain cells by interfering with the brain's circulation. This can lead to memory loss, difficulty concentrating, and confusion and may even accelerate Alzheimer's disease. Saturated fats are also really bad fats and are solid by nature. They are contained in all animal products, meats, and in eggs and whole-milk dairy products. They are also contained in some plant tropical oils (palm kernel, coconut, and cocoa butter). These fats raise your bad LDL cholesterol and lower your good HDL cholesterol. The Diet Fit-Step Plan will lower your bad LDL cholesterol and increase your good HDL cholesterol by following a low total fat diet and walking daily.

II. Unsaturated Fats

1. **Monounsaturated fats** (neutral fats) may actually help to increase the good HDL cholesterol level, and, therefore, they have been found to be cardio-protective. These fats contain **omega-3 fatty acids** which are extremely important in decreasing your risk of heart disease, degenerative diseases of aging and certain forms of cancer. These fats are usually liquid at room temperature and tend to harden or cloud when refrigerated. They are the primary fats found in olive oil, canola oil, peanut oil, most nuts and seeds, avocados and some whole grain products. You should cook with monounsaturated oils such as olive oil, canola oil, or peanut oil. And you should eat monounsaturated foods such as nuts and avocados. These are the **best of all the fats** and are considered to be heart-protective.

2. **Polyunsaturated fats** (essential fatty acids) are always of vegetable origin and are liquid oils. Safflower oil is the highest in polyunsaturates of all oils. Sunflower oil is second, followed by corn oil, sesame seed oil, soybean oil, cottonseed oil, walnut oil and linseed oil. Polyunsaturated fats in limited amounts may help to lower the bad LDL cholesterol level by assisting the body to eliminate excessive amounts of newly manufactured cholesterol. It is essential that you substitute monounsaturated and polyunsaturated fats for saturated fats to maximize their cholesterol-lowering effect. It is interesting to note that we can manufacture saturated fat and most monounsaturated fats in our bodies. Polyunsaturated fats, however, must be

obtained from the diet and are, therefore, called **omega-6 essential fatty acids**. However, polyunsaturated vegetable oils, which are found in margarine, salad dressings, corn oil and processed foods, contain omega-6 fatty acids. These are also considered bad fats when excessive amounts are consumed, since they can set up chronic inflammation in brain tissue, which could lead to brain damage, strokes and degenerative brain diseases like Alzheimer's disease. Therefore, polyunsaturated oils should be limited to 1½ tsp. daily. Otherwise these are considered to be good fats in moderation. Polyunsaturated fats are the good fats when eaten in moderation, but can turn bad when eaten in excess because of their omega-6 fatty acids that can cause inflammation in the body. Here we have an example of a good fat turned bad.

3. **Trans-fats** are fats that have hydrogen atoms added by either heat or pressure. They are formed when hydrogen atoms are added to oils containing mono or polyunsaturated fats. The hydrogenation process converts liquid oils into a more solid form. They then become hydrogenated (solid) or partially hydrogenated (semi-solid) oils and are *very bad fats*. They can increase your risk of heart disease by raising your bad LDL cholesterol and decreasing your good HDL cholesterol. They also have been reported to release a chemical called *Tumor Necrosis Factor*, which can cause inflammation in the body, thus increasing the risk for heart attacks, diabetes, high blood pressure and cancer. They are found in cooking oils, shortening, margarine, many processed and baked foods, cookies, crackers, snack foods, and non-dairy creamers. Always check food labels for hydrogenated or partially hydrogenated oils, which are actually trans-fats.

How Trans Fats Increase Your Weight

1. Ordinarily, when carbohydrates are eaten they are absorbed from the intestinal tract and converted to glucose in the bloodstream. This glucose is absorbed into the body's cells for the production of energy and some of it is stored in the liver and muscles as a form of stored energy called *glycogen*. Glycogen remains in the liver and muscles for future use in the production of energy. When fats are consumed, however, some of them are converted into *fatty acids* in the bloodstream. Fatty acids are readily incorporated into muscle and fat cells throughout the body. Normally fatty acids in muscle cells can be used by the muscle cell membranes for the production of energy by converting fatty acids into glucose. Also these fatty acids help the muscle cells absorb and utilize blood glucose for the production of energy.

2. Trans fats are also absorbed into the muscle cell membrane; however, they negatively affect the muscle cell's ability to absorb glucose from the bloodstream and its ability to convert it into a useful form of energy. When these active muscle cells can not absorb and metabolize glucose, blood sugar levels spike and subsequently cause spikes in blood insulin levels. These increased levels of insulin cause fat to be stored in the body's fat cells since they can not get inside the metabolically active muscle cells. Again, this excess accumulation of fat inside the body's fat cells results in rapid weight gain and subsequent obesity, especially if the consumption of trans fats continues.

3. Trans fats can block the production of the appetite suppressant hormones and mood relaxing hormones such as *serotonin, dopamine* and *nor-epinephrine*. These toxic fats accomplish this nefarious deed by causing the cells in your brain to become inflamed. This inflammatory process results in an increased appetite and food craving and the subsequent increase in the consumption of excess calories. This toxic

process also contributes to anxiety and insomnia. People tend to eat more bad carbs when they can not fall asleep causing additional fat to be stored in your body's fat cells.

4. Trans fats also cause you to gain more belly fat by redistributing stored fatty acids from various locations throughout the body and sending them into the abdominal fat cells. This increase in belly fat is thought to occur because trans fats produce a toxic reaction in the body's fat cells. This reaction forces fat globules into the bloodstream and relocates them into the omentum (a curtain of fat cells lining the abdominal organs). This omentum is located in the middle of the body and in the direct path of these traveling fat globules. Since there are so many fat cells located in the omentum, it is like a large fish net that catches all of these migrating fat cells and stores them as abdominal fat.

How to Elminate Dietary Trans Fats

1. By limiting your total fat intake to no more than 35 grams daily, you will be naturally eliminating most trans-fats from your diet. Stick with healthy monounsaturated fats, which will raise your good HDL cholesterol and lower your bad LDL cholesterol by limiting your total fat intake.

2. Always check labels, even if the label claims to be trans fat-free and make sure all of the fat ingredients on the label add up to the number of grams of total fat listed on the label. If the the amounts of the saturated fat and unsaturated fat don't equal the amount of total fat on the label, then you can be sure that there are hidden trans fats left unlisted.

3. Instead of using any type of vegetable shortening or spreads or margarine, substitute Smart Balance®, Benecol®, Take Control® or Crisco Trans Fat-Free® and Promise® spreads. These new spreads contain healthy monounsaturated fats. Many of these newer spreads also contain heart-healthy omega-3 fatty acids.

4. Frozen dinners, although frozen, still have hydrogenated or partially hydrogenated vegetable oils to preserve their freshness before microwaving.

5. Avoid packaged and processed foods (cakes, cookies, mixes and desserts) since almost all contain trans fats. Even so-called health or protein bars which state "no trans fats" have partially hydrogenated oils as one of their ingredients. Avoid these and look for snacks or health bars that do not contain these trans fats. Powdered cake and cookie mixes usually contain trans fats since they stay fresh for many months before adding water to prepare.

6. Avoid fried foods and fast food restaurants since almost all have some form of partially hydrogenated oils in their products. Avoid most processed deli meats since they contain hydrogenated vegetable oils in addition to carcinogenic nitrates.

7. Restaurants of any kind, including fast food restaurants, are a major source of trans fats. Unfortunately, the FDA has made restaurants exempt from labeling foods for trans fats. Here as elsewhere, like at home, it is important to choose fresh fruits and vegetables, whole grain products, lean protein (fish, fowl and lean meats) and non-fat dairy products in order to avoid trans fats. When dining in a restaurant, ask if the desserts are made on the premises. These desserts are less likely to contain trans fats than those desserts that have been mass produced at outside food processing companies and bakeries.

8. When dining out, request that your food be either broiled, steamed, or grilled. These preparations are less likely to contain trans fats. There are many new restaurants that have taken the initiative to limit trans fats in their foods.

9. There are many foods and compounds which help to eliminate trans fats from the body. These include the omega-3 fatty acids which are present in fish oils and flaxseeds. These healthy fatty acids help to produce a compound called *cholecystokinin* which helps to decrease hunger and helps to counteract the adverse effects of fatty acids on the intestinal tract and liver.

Also, citrus foods such as oranges, limes and lemons contain the antioxidant vitamin C, which helps to eliminate free radicals which occur from the ingestion of fatty acids. Vitamin C rich diets help the liver's ability to break down trans fats and eliminate them from the body.

10. Vegetables such as Brussels sprouts, broccoli, cabbage and cauliflower are known as cruciferous vegetables. They contain compounds called *sulforaphane* and *indole-3 carbinol* which help to eliminate trans fats from the intestinal tract and help the liver's ability to convert these trans fats into water soluble components which can be easily eliminated by the intestinal tract. Several fruits contain phytochemicals called *anthocyanins* which are found in papaya, guava, kiwi and cranberries. These rich and powerful phytochemicals can cause the elimination of trans fats from the body, particularly if these fruits are consumed as juices. The anthocyanin rich fruits which are contained in juices can combine with the trans fats and eliminate them from the intestinal tract.

SAY NO-NO TO YO-YO DIETS

The Framingham Heart Study, which has followed more than 5,000 people for almost 40 years, recently indicated a health hazard for chronic dieters. People who lost 10% of their body weight had an almost 20% reduction in the incidence of heart disease. So what's the problem? These same dieters, who gained back the 10% of their body weight, raised their heart disease risk by almost 30%. So if you weigh 160 lbs. and lost 10% or 16 lbs., you decreased your heart disease risk by 20%. But if you gained back that 16 lbs., you increased your risk of heart attack by 30%, an overall net gain of 10% and you still weigh the same 160 lbs. Sounds scary to me, folks! How many times have you heard the old saying that "I've lost enough weight over the years to equal two or three whole persons and I've gained every bit of it back?" Yo-yo dieting or weight-cycling makes it harder to permanently lose weight and is much more dangerous to your health.

Experts in the fields of physiology, biochemistry, psychology, nutrition and medicine have come up with the following startling findings about yo-yo dieting:

1. The **weight-loss/weight-gain cycle** actually increases your desire for fatty foods. Animal research studies at Yale University showed that rats that had lost weight rapidly on low-calorie diets always chose more fat in their diets when given a choice between fat, protein, and carbohydrates. These rats always put on more weight than when they started and in a much shorter time than it had taken them to lose the weight.

2. **Yo-yo dieters increase the percentage of body fat** to lean body tissue with repeated bouts of weight gain and loss. People who lose weight rapidly on a low carbohydrate, high-fat diet can lose a significant amount of muscle tissue. If the weight is regained again, they usually regain more fat and less muscle because it is easier for the body to gain fat than it is to rebuild muscle tissue.

3. **Body fat gets redistributed in the abdomen from the thighs, buttocks and hips** after weight cycling. Medical research has definitely shown that fat deposits above the waist increases the risk of heart disease and diabetes, not to mention an unsightly paunch.

4. When you lose weight by cutting calories, your **basal metabolic rate (BMR)** slows down, because it is the body's defense mechanism against starvation. The body can't tell the difference between starvation and low calorie dieting; consequently, your body is trying to conserve energy by burning fewer calories. This is the reason it becomes harder to lose weight after a week or two, even though you are eating exactly the same amount of calories as you did when you first started your diet. This slow-down in the basal metabolic rate (BMR) persists even after the diet is over and accounts for the rapid-rebound, excessive weight gain that always happens to the dieter when they go off their diet. This slow-down in metabolic rate can occur even after a single attempt at dieting.

However, the repeated effects of weight-cycling diets can affect the basal metabolic rate (BMR) much more, making additional weight-loss almost impossible and rebound weight gain almost inevitable. The yo-yo dieter is often heard to say—"I'm heavier now than I was before I started this diet."

5. An enzyme called **lipoprotein lipase (LPL)** becomes more active when you cut calories. This enzyme controls the amount of fat that is stored in your body's fat cells. Dieting, therefore, makes the body more efficient at storing fat, which is exactly the opposite of what a dieter wants. As you reduce your calorie intake, the enzyme LPL starts to activate the fat-storing process. This is another defense mechanism that the body uses to prevent starvation. Remember, the enzyme LPL doesn't know that you are dieting; it thinks that you are starving to death.

6. Women and men dieters who've lost a substantial amount of weight were compared to a group of normal weight people. After they lost weight, the previously obese individuals required surprisingly fewer calories to maintain their weight than the normal-weight women. In this study, obese people who lost weight needed only 2000 calories a day to maintain their weight (125 lbs.) compared to 2300 calories per day to maintain the exact same weight (125 lbs.) by normal-weight people. Who said dieting was fair?

7. Chronic dieters who exhibited repeated cycles of weight gain and weight loss showed an increased risk of sudden death from heart attacks, according to a recent medical report. This study followed 1500 women over a period of 25 years who had engaged in cyclic-dieting.

Say Yes-Yes to Walking

We know that losing weight lowers blood pressure, reduces the risk of heart disease, lowers blood cholesterol and triglycerides and increases the HDL ("good" cholesterol). The answer is that dieting alone is not the best way to lose and maintain weight. The following is a list of the reasons why walking is the only safe and effective method to lose and maintain your ideal body weight:

1. **Exercise, particularly walking**, is the real answer to preventing the weight loss/weight-gain cycle from occurring. Walking makes it less likely you'll gain the weight back again because you lose more fat and less muscle tissue with exercise. Also, walking prevents the slow-down in basal metabolic rate that always occurs with a yo-yo diet. Actually walking slightly **increases the BMR,** which helps to burn calories at a faster rate. Walking also **reduces the production of the enzyme lipoprotein lipase (LPL)**, which in turn decreases the amount of fat stored in the fat cells.

2. Walking also regulates the brain's appetite controller, the **appestat**. The more you walk, the more you decrease the appestat's hunger mechanism. Inactivity, on the other hand, stimulates the appetite control mechanism to make you hungry.

3. Walking, by increasing the aerobic metabolism of the body, **redirects the stomach's blood supply** to the exercising muscles, which in turn decreases your appetite.

4. And finally, walking encourages the body to *burn fat rather than carbohydrates*. This enables the body's blood sugar to stay at a relatively constant normal level. When the brain's blood sugar is normal we are not hungry. Both strenuous exercise and low-calorie dieting, however, burn carbohydrates rather than fats, causing a sharp drop in the blood sugar. When the brain's blood sugar drops as it does in dieting or strenuous exercises, then we feel hungry in order to counteract this low blood sugar. The high fiber content of the Diet Fit-Step Mystery Plan also controls the body's appetite center, making overeating high-fat calories next to impossible.

POWER BREAKFAST WITHOUT THE FAT

Eating a healthy breakfast of complex carbohydrates (whole grain cereals and fruits) and lean protein (egg white, low-fat milk or yogurt) combined with a morning walk will boost your metabolic rate all morning long after you have finished your breakfast and your walk. Skipping breakfast, on the other hand, decreases your basal metabolic rate and leads to mid-morning snacking of refined sugars (cakes, donuts, etc.) and coffee to feel your energy level boost.

Dietary fat, which is found in most processed foods, only uses up five calories out of every 100 fat calories consumed during the digestive process. Eating complex carbohydrates (fruits, vegetables, whole grain cereals, and nuts) uses up almost 25 calories out of every 1,000 calories consumed during the digestive process. So it is quite evident that complex carbohydrates increase your post meal metabolic rate by burning more of the calories consumed during the digestive process. You are in effect burning some of the calories that you are eating rather than absorbing all of them into your body. A high fat, high refined carbohydrate breakfast (bacon, eggs, potatoes, and white bread) on the other hand, literally sticks the fat to your ribs. Also, many types of granola cereals are usually high in fats and sugars and should be avoided as a breakfast cereal, unless their ingredients indicate that they are low in fat and sugar and have high fiber content (5 or more grams).

BOOST YOUR FAT-BURNING METABOLISM

1. You will burn more calories if you eat **small, frequent meals** or snack every three to four hours. Eating small, frequent meals helps keep the body's insulin level more even, which makes it less likely you will store fat. If you go for a long period between large meals, your insulin levels spike, which makes it more likely you will store the extra calories and sugar as fat. This is because sporadic surges in insulin levels cause more sugar to be stored in your body's cells as fat, rather than being used as a source of fuel to produce energy.

2. People who eat a skimpy breakfast or no breakfast at all and very little lunch save up all of their calories for a big meal at dinner. This is probably the worst way to burn fat and the best way to store fat because of the inefficient utilization of glucose as a fuel. Instead **glucose gets turned into fat stores** in the body's cells.

3. If you eat every few hours you will have more energy because sugar will be used efficiently as **fuel to produce energy**. On the other hand, if you eat infrequently or wait until you are famished, then you will be fatigued because the sugar will not be able to be used as fuel efficiently, and energy production will go down.

    a. Your brain needs **fuel to produce energy** to enable you to think clearly, concentrate, and to work efficiently. Also your body needs fuel to help you exercise for longer periods of time, and to move faster and more efficiently. This steady supply of fuel can only be accomplished by a steady supply of glucose being utilized to produce the energy required for proper brain and body function.

    b. **So the formula is:** small, frequent, high fiber, lean protein, low-fat complex carbohydrate meals = steady level of insulin = constant supply of glucose = production of energy to boost body and mind functions.

4. It is important to have **a snack** (piece of fruit or a small amount of whole grain cereal or a slice of whole grain bread) before your walking exercise workout (with or without weights), in order to increase your production of energy. Exercise stabilizes insulin and glucose levels, so that energy production is maximized. The combination of exercise and a small helpful snack improves your energy level.

5. On the Diet Fit-Step Plan, the addition of **lean protein** (lean meats, white meat of chicken or turkey, fish, non-fat dairy products including soy and egg whites, whole grains and bran, nuts and seeds) all contribute to burning fat calories and boosting energy. Protein suppresses your appetite and produces the necessary fuel for the production of energy for all of your body's

needs. Protein is made up of amino acids, which are essential for your cells' metabolism and for the repair and maintenance of all of your body's cells.

6. Several recent research studies have confirmed that people, who consume two to three servings of **calcium containing foods** such as milk, cheese, or yogurt daily, lost considerably more weight than those individuals who just reduced their calorie intake, while consuming very little in the way of dairy products.

   a. High calcium diets have been proven to inhibit the production of a certain calcium-regulating hormone *calcitrol*, so that the amount of calcium and fat stored in the body's cells actually decreases. This actually causes you to store less fat, and ultimately lose more weight. On the other hand, it has been shown that low calcium diets actually increase this calcium-regulating hormone, which causes both calcium and fat to be stored in the body's cells and ultimately causes weight to be gained.

   b. This calcium-regulating hormone works in conjunction with the protein found in dairy products to burn fat more efficiently and more quickly, which is another reason dairy products help you to lose weight. Research studies have also shown that low-fat dairy products have the same ability to limit fat storage and burn fat calories, as does whole milk dairy products. So non-fat milk, yogurt, and low-fat cheeses are ideal for a weight reduction program.

   c. Newer research has shown that people burn more fat in their abdominal region (waist circumference), and subsequently lose more inches by combining two to three low-fat dairy products a day with a high fiber, low-fat diet. This reduction in abdominal fat can help to decrease the risk of diabetes, high blood pressure, heart disease, and a condition known as the metabolic syndrome (high blood pressure, diabetes, obesity, coronary artery disease). For people who are lactose intolerant, lactose-free milk and yogurt work just as well.

Metabolic Syndrome: Fit or Fat?

In a recent study reported at the Third World Congress on *insulin resistance syndrome*, it was shown that a patient's fitness level is as important as obesity in the development of the metabolic syndrome, as well as in all causes of mortality. People with low levels of cardiovascular and cardio-respiratory fitness and those with low levels of muscular strength were prone to develop the metabolic syndrome to a greater degree than those patients who were just obese. The metabolic syndrome is defined as a condition that is composed of diabetes, high blood pressure, obesity, high lipids, and cardiovascular disease. This appears to result from the patient's inability to process and utilize insulin effectively.

It has been previously thought that obesity was the major factor in the development of the metabolic syndrome; however, it has been recently discovered that low levels of fitness also contribute to the development of this syndrome. Patients with moderate to high levels of cardiovascular fitness were found to be significantly less likely to develop the metabolic syndrome than were those individuals with low fitness levels. This study suggested that a patient's low level of fitness may be more important than his/her obesity in determining his/her risk for developing the metabolic syndrome. Improved muscular strength was shown to decrease an individual's likelihood of developing the metabolic syndrome, possibly because of the muscles ability to process insulin and sugar more effectively.

Metabolic Syndrome Warning Signs

1. Waist size greater than:
   36 inches for women and 42 inches for men
2. Blood pressure over 140/90
3. HDL cholesterol less than 50 in women and less than 40 in men
4. LDL cholesterol more than 100 in either men or women
5. Cholesterol levels over 200
6. Triglyceride levels over 160

Melt Belly Fat

Refined carbohydrates that we eat are gradually absorbed into the bloodstream, which causes a sudden spike in insulin production. This excess amount of insulin in our blood causes these digested refined carbohydrates to head straight into our fat cells, particularly our belly fat cells, since the abdominal or belly fat cells are the closest to the digestive tract and contain the most concentrated amounts of fat cells in the entire body. Once the excess insulin has done its work by lowering the blood sugar and packing fat into the fat cells of the abdomen, the low blood sugar that results causes another round of carbohydrate cravings. It is a "lose-lose combination."

As we age, we crave more carbohydrates, and the more carbs we eat, the more calories become stored as fat in our abdomen. Due to certain hormonal changes that regulate our digestive system, we become less able to burn carbs for fuel, thus making carbs more likely to become stored as fat in the body, particularly in the abdomen. This becomes a vicious cycle since the more carbs we store as belly fat, the more carbohydrates we crave in our diet. Stored abdominal fat suppresses the formation of fat-burning hormones such as *leptin* which helps to keep blood sugars steady. Consequently, the more abdominal fat you store makes it easier for you to gain more weight.

If you can lose abdominal fat, you will diminish carbohydrate cravings and subsequently lose the unwanted belly fat. By eating high fiber foods you can actually block the absorption of refined carbohydrates and starches. This is accomplished by the increased fiber foods preventing the absorption of these refined carbohydrates by forming a web or net of fibers that encircles or tangles up these starches and carries them out of the digestive tract, almost completely intact and undigested. By blocking most of the absorption of these refined starches, less sugar and insulin are present in the bloodstream, which subsequently results in fewer cravings for carbohydrates. Less craving for carbs results in more belly fat being burned and more weight being lost, particularly around the abdomen.

High fiber foods, particularly beans (white, kidney, fava and pinto beans) contain an enzyme-blocking compound which blocks pancreatic enzymes (amylase and lipase) from breaking down refined starches. By inhibiting these enzymes from absorbing refined carbohydrates, your digestive tract bypasses absorption of these starches and transports them out of your digestive tract as though they were never totally digested. This results in a much slower rise in blood sugar, which in turns does not cause a spike in insulin production and consequently reduces your craving for carbohydrates.

BELLY FAT MELTING TIPS

1. **THE FIBER-MINERAL COMBO** – foods that contain both fiber and the mineral magnesium help to decrease the risk of developing the so-called *metabolic syndrome*. This syndrome consists of high blood pressure, diabetes, high blood fats, particularly triglycerides, insulin resistance, obesity and a tendency to accumulate excess amounts of abdominal fat. The combination of magnesium and fiber prevents sudden spikes in blood sugar and blood insulin levels that cause excess amounts of fat to become stored in your body's abdominal fat cells. Foods rich in magnesium include peas, beans (lima and kidney beans), avocados, spinach, broccoli, whole grains, wheat germ, brown rice, sweet potatoes with skin and many fruits.

2. **LOW-FAT DAIRY PRODUCTS (CHEESE, MILK, YOGURT)** – these low-fat dairy products suppress the hormone *calcitrol* that causes fat to be stored in your abdominal fat cells. These low-fat dairy products also reduce the risk of developing the metabolic syndrome by up to 50%. Also, the combination of calcium and protein in these daily products combine to burn additional calories and help in weight-loss.

3. **TRANS FATS** – Trans fats can almost double your risk of developing the metabolic syndrome. These fats are either hydrogenated or partially hydrogenated oils that are found in margarine, fast and frozen foods, baked goods, non-dairy creamers

and most packaged and processed foods. These fats can raise your blood pressure and increase your blood sugar, and therefore, block your arteries with cholesterol deposits. Recent research has shown that every 3 to 5% increase in the consumption of trans fats results in a 2 pound weight gain every four to six weeks, particularly around the abdominal wall.

4. **AVOID STRESS** – You can avoid stress by meditating, walking, doing yoga or any activity that you find calming. Stress unfortunately causes the body to produce the stress hormone *cortisol* which can increase your blood fats, particularly the triglycerides, and also increases your blood pressure and blood sugar. This deadly combination increases your risk of developing insulin resistance, which subsequently produces more belly fat, and thus, increases the risk of developing the metabolic syndrome. Recent studies have shown that reducing cortisol production by engaging in calming activities and exercise helps to prevent the development of the metabolic syndrome with all of its attendant hazards including excess storage of belly fat.

5. **THE MEDITERRANEAN DIET** – The Mediterranean diet consists primarily of fruits, vegetables, whole grains, nuts, seafood, olive oil and small amounts of lean meats. This diet can actually reduce the risk of developing the metabolic syndrome by up to 50%. The diet improves blood sugar and insulin control and reduces blood pressure simply by increasing the intake of plant foods. The monounsaturated heart-healthy olive oil helps to decrease blood pressure, blood sugar, obesity, blood fats, coronary artery disease, cancer and degenerative diseases. This diet increases the level of good HDL cholesterol by more than 30% which acts to clear out cholesterol deposits in blocked arteries, thus decreasing the risk of heart attacks and strokes.

The Case of the Unwanted Pounds

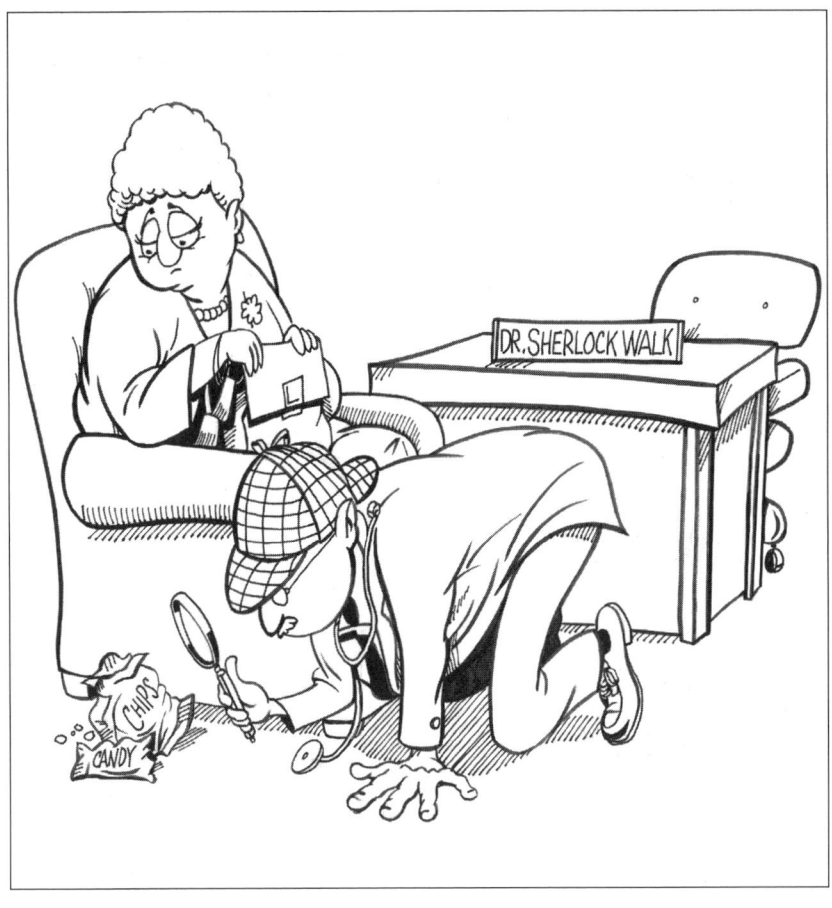

5

Dr. Walk's Mystery Diet Clues

The *Diet Fit-Step Mystery Plan* consists of a series of weight-loss and fitness clues, which are published regularly in my on-line publication entitled, *Dr. Walk's Diet & Fitness Newsletter*. I have shared these diet, fitness and health tips with my patients over the past 15 to 20 years, many of whom have followed them regularly with excellent weight-loss and fitness results. I have included many of these clues in this new book and I hope that you will share all of the weight-loss, fitness and good health benefits that my patients have enjoyed over the past two decades. By following the Diet Fit-Step Mystery Plan, you will *permanently lose all of those unwanted pounds* that have plagued you for a lifetime.

MYSTERY WEIGHT-LOSS FACTS

1. **Nuts** are packed with nutrition. They contain vitamin E, B-complex, folic acid, fiber, omega-3 fatty acids, and arginine (an amino acid). These nutrients contained in nuts have been shown to prevent heart disease and strokes and protect the heart against irregular heart rhythms and help to maintain your blood vessels' natural elasticity. The monounsaturated fats contained in nuts also have other heart-protective properties. These monounsaturated can lower blood cholesterol, particularly the bad LDL cholesterol, which can lead to coronary

artery disease and they can also help to reduce blood pressure. Frequent consumption of nuts (four to five servings per week) has been shown to reduce the risk of coronary heart disease by as much as 50%. Nuts also have been shown to decrease both the total cholesterol by 5-10% and the LDL cholesterol by 15-20%.

Nuts are also packed with protein, which is good for you and acts as a natural appetite suppressant by the very nature of its slow digestion and subsequent absorption into the bloodstream. Almost all of the energy contained in the protein you eat is burned as fuel for your body's metabolic functions; therefore, hardly any of the calories contained in dietary protein are converted into fat storage. The protein content of nuts satisfies your hunger mechanism quickly so that you consume fewer calories. A study published in *The Journal of Nutrition* indicated that of all edible plants, *walnuts* have one of the highest concentrations of antioxidants. In a more recent study reported in the *Journal of Circulation*, from the Hospital Clinic of Barcelona, Spain, Dr. Emilio Ros said that, "This is the first time a whole food, not its isolated components, has shown this beneficial effect on vascular health." He further stated that, "Walnuts differ from all other nuts because of their high content of *alpha-linolenic acid* (ALA), a plant-based omega-3 fatty acid, which may provide additional heart-protective properties."

Several other beneficial components of walnuts include: L-arginine, which may be cardio-protective by dilating the arteries, and fiber, folic acid, gamma-tocopherol, and other antioxidants, which also help to prevent atherosclerosis (hardening of the arteries). Nuts, particularly walnuts and almonds, which are rich in monounsaturated fats, cause the brain to release a hormone called *cholecystokinin*, which actually shuts down the appetite control mechanism in the brain and prevents hunger. Two ounces of almonds is enough to release this appetite-suppressing hormone. Remember that nuts are also high in fat; however, they contain the heart-healthy monounsaturated fats which have been shown to have both health benefits and weight reduction properties. Nuts are packed full of nutrition. They contain folic acid, vitamin D, copper, magnesium, fiber, and healthy monounsaturated fats. You just have to be careful to limit the amount of nuts that you eat in order to stay under the 35 grams of total fat per day on the Diet Fit-Step Plan.

2. Three to four ounces of **red wine** every other day is heart-healthy, since the red grapes contain *resveratrol*, a super antioxidant which helps to prevent strokes, blood clots, hypertension and heart disease, providing that you have no underlying liver or cardiac problems which prevents consumption of any alcoholic beverages. You can get the same benefits by eating red grapes or purple grape juice without the alcohol and the fruit sugar content of wine and grapes helps to satisfy your appetite.

3. **Chocolate**, particularly dark chocolate, contains healthful nutrients called flavonoids. These flavonoids are effective antioxidants that can protect your heart from dangerous free radicals that can damage heart cells. Dark chocolate has been shown to have proven health benefits because it contains at least 70-75% cocoa. It also contains health promoting antioxidants (polyphenols and resveratrol), which can reduce the risk of blood clots that can cause strokes and heart attacks These flavonoids also protect you from heart disease by decreasing the LDL bad cholesterol and increasing the HDL good cholesterol in the body. These antioxidants also produce an enzyme called *endothelial nitric oxide synthase (ENOS),* which relaxes the blood vessels thus lowering your blood pressure. Dark chocolate also has been shown to be a mood lifter, as well as a blood pressure lowering agent.

Chocolate however, is loaded with sugar, fat and calories, which can contribute to weight gain. Dark chocolate contains less sugar than milk or white chocolate; however, it still is high in calories and saturated fat, so enjoy your dark chocolate as long as you don't eat more than 1½ ounces per day. Chocolate is a great appetite suppressant, since it easily satisfies your appetite with just a small amount of its sweet taste.

4. **A high-protein** dietary intake appears to have a blood pressure lowering effect, particularly when consuming vegetable protein rather than animal protein. Also the unique combination of protein and calcium in non-fat or low-fat dairy products helps to keep your appetite satisfied for a relatively long period of time. Also, this calcium and protein combination found in dairy products appears to increase the metabolic rate and burn fat calories faster.

5. Drinking lots of **water** helps to satisfy your hunger mechanism by filling you up either before or during a meal. The water will help you eat less at each meal, since your stomach will not know whether it's food or water that's in your stomach. Drinking six, 8 oz. glasses of water a day is a great way to keep your appetite satisfied and help you lose weight. Water is one of the best diet foods, since it contains no calories and satisfies your hunger quickly. Water also fuels your body's energy level, since all of the body's metabolic processes require a constant supply of water to function efficiently.

6. **Food cravings** are a constant battle in the war against overeating. When you're under stress or anxious, you have a tendency to crave high calorie foods and sweets. You can overcome food cravings by eating low calorie, crunchy foods such as celery, carrots, apples, rice cakes, popcorn, nuts, seeds and low-fat pretzels. The crunch factor helps to reduce stress and anxiety by relaxing your tense neck and facial muscles. Fruits are also a great way to combat sweet food cravings. Also, lean protein and low-fat, high fiber foods produce good-feeling hormones (endorphins and serotonin), which help to prevent you from giving in to food cravings for sweets and high fat foods.

7. **Fish oils** contained in fatty fish are also low in total saturated fat and calories and satisfy your appetite easily due to the lean protein content. The fish oils contained in fish such as salmon, tuna, and haddock contain *omega-3 fatty acids*, which have been recently found to improve exercise-induced asthma. These omega-3 fatty acids appear to reduce the risk of

heart disease, hypertension, strokes, blood clots, degenerative diseases of aging and some forms of cancer. There are also omega-3 fatty acids present in plant foods, such as walnuts and in flaxseed. These are known as ALA (alpha-linolenic acid). The body, however, must convert ALA into DHA and EPA in order to have the same health benefits as with eating fish. Fish are low in calories and total saturated fats and are essential for an effective weight reduction program. Eat fish three to four times per week, whether at home or in a restaurant, for a healthy, low-fat, high-protein, great diet tip.

8. **Calcium burns fat and builds bones:** Several new studies have shown that people who regularly drink skim milk and eat yogurt or have one serving of low-fat cheese per day, lose an average of 1½ pounds per month, with no additional change in their diets. It is believed that calcium decreases the stores of fat in the fat cells by actually burning stored fat. Also, it is thought that the protein content in milk, yogurt and cheese replaces the fat stored in the fat cells by a unique process of providing extra protein to the body's cells. This combination of calcium and protein which is present in milk, yogurt and cheese helps the body to burn fat and store protein.

   If you consume low amounts of calcium-rich dairy foods, your body produces a calcium regulating hormone called *calcitrol,* which acts by causing the body to push calcium in your bloodstream into your fat cells. This storage of calcium in your fat cells causes the body to burn less fat, thus, making more fat available to be deposited in your fat cells and subsequently weight is gained. High calcium diets have been proven to inhibit the production of this calcium-regulating hormone, so that the amount of calcium and fat stored in the body's cells actually decreases. This actually causes you to store less fat, and ultimately lose more weight. Newer research has even shown that by combining two to three low-fat dairy products a day with a reduced calorie intake, people burn more fat in their abdominal region (waist circumference), and subsequently lose more inches.

9. **Detective D,** known commonly as vitamin D, has been linked to a myriad of health benefits. Vitamin D has been shown to increase the amount of calcium in the bones of your body. New studies have shown that excessive calcium buildup in your arteries can increase your risk of heart disease. However, when calcium is combined with vitamin D, calcium is forced into your bones rather than into your arteries. This absorption of calcium into your bones helps to prevent osteoporosis by strengthening the structure of the bones and supporting muscles. Calcium also aids in the lessening of many forms of arthritis. The combination of Vitamin D and calcium also act as an effective appetite suppressant.

   It has been shown that more than 50% of people have low levels of Vitamin D. Vitamin D may protect against arthritis, osteoporosis, heart disease and strokes, Parkinson's disease, dementia, Alzheimer's disease, multiple sclerosis, tuberculosis, psoriasis, fatigue, upper respiratory viruses including the flu (worse in the winter when sunlight and Vitamin D are at there lowest), and certain forms of cancer including ovarian, prostate, kidney, and colon cancers. The active ingredient in vitamin D is *Calciferol* or Vitamin D3, which appears to slow or inhibit the growth of cancer cells.

10. **Avoid sugary sodas, teas, juices, and sports drinks.** Use fresh orange juice, grapefruit juice, vegetable or tomato juice (low sodium), and non-caffeinated teas, coffee and diet sodas. Cream, whole milk, or powdered creamers should be avoided in coffee or tea and you should substitute skim milk or non-fat dairy creams. Avoid drinking a lot of artificially sweetened drinks as they can increase your appetite, due to the hypoglycemic effect (it lowers your blood sugar). Also, avoid the so-called sports drinks, which contain both sugar and caffeine. These drinks instead of hydrating you can actually cause dehydration and may in fact raise your blood pressure and cause insulin spikes, which can result in weight gain, not weight-loss. Always make plain water (tap or bottled) your drink of choice.

Mystery Diet Clues

WHAT TO THINK ABOUT BEFORE EATING:

1. Before food shopping, prepare a list and only go to the market after you've eaten. Going to the market when hungry can lead to impulse purchases of high fat snack foods. Buy only those items on your list. Don't deviate from this list with snack foods, which you might have a tendency to buy, if you had not eaten prior to shopping.

2. When shopping for packaged or canned goods, make sure the item of food you are purchasing has no more than 1.5 – 2.0 grams of total fat per serving. If it is higher, compare other brands. Always look for non-fat or low-fat products; however, read the fat content on the nutritional label, and don't depend on a label that says "low-fat food." Many so-called low-fat items are fairly high in total fat content; for example 2% milk has 5 grams of fat, and 98% fat free yogurt can have 3.5 to 4 grams of total fat. Always choose foods that are less than 2.0 grams of total fat. Also watch out for labels that say "cholesterol-free." These foods may have 0 grams of cholesterol; however, they may contain many grams of total fat.

3. Foods should be kept out of sight, in your refrigerator or pantry, between meals. Do not place serving dishes on the table during meals to reduce temptation to take second helpings.

4. Don't skip meals. Skipping meals lowers your blood sugar, which brings on cravings for high-carbohydrate, high calorie foods. Eating 3-4, or even 5, small meals per day is far better than eating one or two large meals. When your blood sugar remains constant, you are less likely to overeat. Individuals who skip breakfast usually wind up with a high fat, high-sugar snack mid-morning, like a coffee break with a doughnut. A high fiber, low-fat cereal with fruit and skim milk for breakfast will hold you comfortably until lunchtime.

5. Eat meals more slowly. Take smaller, less frequent bites and

chew each mouthful for a longer period of time. Pause between each section of the meal. If you are still hungry when you are finished your first portion, wait at least 15 minutes to see whether or not you really want more. Leave the table as soon as you are finished eating and spend less time in the kitchen or areas that remind you of eating.

6. Restrict your meals to one or two locations in the home for eating to avoid eating in every room. This will reduce the tendency to snack during the day.

7. Don't use food as a stress reliever. People have a tendency to seek out high-fat, high-sugar foods when under stress. Substitute music, reading, walking, meditation or a warm bath for food cravings.

8. Don't start a weight reduction program just prior to the holiday season or before vacation time, since these are the most unsuccessful times to begin this type of project. The most important part of any successful diet is starting it. Once you've made up your mind to begin your diet, you're halfway there. You must be ready from the very beginning to discipline yourself. Just like every other part of your life, discipline is a must!

9. If you order in, don't eat out of the container, like when you order Chinese food, otherwise you'll eat the whole portion. Put the different foods on plates, and eat one half the amount of each food and refrigerate the rest for the next day. If you order a pizza, unless there are several people present, take out one or two slices and refrigerate the rest.

10. If you take lunch to work, take a half of a sandwich and a cup of soup to lunch or a big mixed salad without the dressing. If you eat a snack at home, don't eat out of the container that the food came in, like a bag of chips, pretzels, or a container of ice cream or dessert. Serve a small portion in a bowl, and stop before you feel full.

FOOD SELECTION AND PREPARATION:

1. Eat salad greens and vegetables before the main course since these will take the edge off your hunger for higher calorie meat, poultry and fish portions. Substitute non-fat salad dressings or non-fat mayonnaise for regular varieties of these condiments. If not available, either use no dressing, or keep a small portion of dressing on the side and just dip your fork gently into the dressing every 2-3 bites of salad to get the taste without the added fat calories.

2. Soups and stews can be loaded with hidden fats. Refrigerate them overnight after preparing, and skim off the layer of fat that is lying on the surface of the stew or soup. This will remove more than 75% of the fat contained in these products. Choose soups loaded with vegetables and beans, and avoid any soups that are cream-based.

3. Hot foods, such as soups, and foods that require a lot of chewing will leave you with a greater feeling of satisfaction because they take a longer time to swallow and absorb.

4. Breads that are high in fiber, low in fat are the following: whole grain, bran-enriched, cracked wheat, whole-wheat pita, rye, pumpernickel and those labeled "high fiber breads." Avoid the high fat, low fiber breads like French, Italian, white, garlic bread, rolls and bagels. Remember to check the ingredients label. If the first ingredient doesn't say "whole," then it is not a whole-grain, high fiber bread. Choose whole wheat or oat bran English muffins, whole-wheat rolls or bread, whole wheat or oat bran bagels, instead of sweet rolls, doughnuts, cakes and white bread. Remember to always scoop out the inside of rolls or bagels. Use jelly, honey, fruit preserves and all-fruit jams instead of margarine or butter, as spreads for your breads.

5. Make your meals attractive with colorful foods, garnishes and greens, such as carrots, tomatoes, broccoli, spinach, peppers, yams, celery, and parsley, in order to make them more appealing. Also vary your menu plans daily to avoid boredom.

Remember that the more colorful the foods are, the more phyto-nutrients they contain.

6. Fresh vegetables and fruits are better choices than canned fruits and vegetables, which can be loaded with salt or sugar. Fruits and vegetable skins are excellent sources of fiber, as are the seeds in berries, tomatoes, cucumbers, and pumpkins. Steamed vegetables, with or without herbs, can be cooked in a basket over boiling water. Steaming retains the flavor, color and nutrients of the vegetable.

7. Fresh or canned beans of any variety are excellent sources of fiber and vitamins. Their low-fat content makes them excellent companions to any meal. Make sure they are not prepared with meat (example: baked beans with bacon). Avoid high fat refried beans, but non-fat refried beans are okay.

8. Low-fat, non-fat, or part skim-milk cheeses should be substituted for all other cheeses. Make sure, however, that you check the total fat content per serving size. Non-fat yogurt is an excellent source of calcium and its lactobacillus, and other cultures are friendly bacteria for your colon.

9. Peeling a potato (white or sweet) before cooking or eating removes more than 25% of its nutrients and 35-40% of its fiber. A baked potato is an excellent food for meals or snacks (high fiber, low-fat), compared to French fries, which are saturated with up to 15 grams of fat per serving. However, if you have a craving for French fries, you can prepare low-fat French fries by thinly slicing potatoes, using vegetable non-fat sprays like Pam®, and baking for 20-30 minutes in an oven at approximately 300 degrees, or microwaving for 3 to 5 minutes. Keep your portion size small.

10. If you put salt on poultry, fish or meat before cooking, the food loses a good portion of its vitamin and mineral content during the cooking process. This is because the added salt causes the food to be drained of its nutrients during the cooking process, which end up in the cooking broth.

11. Trim all visible skin and fat from poultry and meat before cooking. Either roast (using a rack), grill or broil meat, poultry and fish. The fat drips off during cooking. Baste with broth or vegetable juice to preserve moisture (defatted chicken broth is a good alternative). Or, a light dusting of olive oil is all that is necessary, and many companies now make olive oil sprays, which use considerably less fat than the tablespoon method. Never use butter, margarine, shortening, or gravy mixes.

12. Non-stick pans use less fat than cast iron, copper or aluminum pans. Use non-stick vegetable sprays as your first choice; otherwise, a small amount of olive oil (1 tsp.) or canola oil can be used for cooking. Stir-frying in a pan or wok is a fast way to make tasty vegetables, chicken, meats or fish. Add very small amounts of olive or peanut oil and seasonings followed by either defatted chicken broth or low-sodium soy sauce.

13. Sautéing: Use non-stick, non-fat vegetable sprays or a small amount of wine or defatted broth. Vegetables, fish, poultry or low-fat meats can be mixed together in a pan. Then add herbs, such as thyme, basil, sage, or dill, for added taste.

14. Microwaving uses the foods' own moisture to cook. It's quick and easy, and you don't have to add any fat when microwaving. Almost all foods are microwaveable.

SNACKS AND DESSERTS:

1. A tasty non-fat dessert is *angel food cake* with fresh fruit and non-fat whipped cream. A slice of cheese or chocolate cake has up to 14 grams of fat. The angel food cake, as described above, has less than 1.5 grams of fat.

2. *Sherbet, sorbet, frozen fruit bars and non-fat frozen yogurts* are excellent substitutes for your ice cream sweet tooth.

3. *Non-fat popcorn* is an excellent low-fat, high fiber snack. Don't add butter or salt. Use hot air popper or microwave non-

fat varieties. Other low-fat snacks include hard pretzels (non-fat), and flavored rice cakes.

4. Excellent fat-free *fruit and veggie* snack-food choices include dried or fresh fruits, raisins, peaches, apples, plums, apricots, bananas, baby carrots, and celery stalks.

5. *Nuts* are packed with nutrition and because of their protein content are very filling. They contain vitamin E, B-complex, folic acid, fiber, omega-3 fatty acids, and arginine (an amino acid). These nutrients contained in nuts have been shown to reduce bad LDL cholesterol and increase good HDL cholesterol and therefore help to reduce the incidence of heart disease and strokes. The nutrients in nuts also protect the heart against irregular heart rhythms and help to maintain your blood vessels' natural elasticity.

6. *Chocolate*, particularly dark chocolate, contains healthful nutrients called flavonoids. These flavonoids are antioxidants that protect your heart from dangerous free radicals that can damage heart cells. These flavonoids also protect you from heart disease by decreasing the LDL bad cholesterol and increasing the HDL good cholesterol in the body. Chocolate also raises blood levels of endorphins (feeling-good hormones), which helps to relax you from anxiety and stress. Also, chocolate is actually good for a weight-loss program, because by just eating a small amount of dark chocolate, your appetite-control mechanism is quickly satisfied. A medium sized dark chocolate peppermint patty has only 2.5 grams of total fat, 1.5 grams of saturated fat, and zero trans-fats and cholesterol.

7. High-fiber, low-fat *cereal and/or granola bars* with real fruit are very filling and satisfying snacks. Just make sure that the sugar, fat, and calorie content is not too high.

8. A *root beer float* is a great satisfying drink to have as a snack. Use diet root beer and non-fat frozen vanilla yogurt in a tall ice cream glass.

9. A *smoothie* made in the blender with all kinds of fruits, frozen non-fat yogurt or non-fat milk, and 1 tsp. of wheat germ, and whey protein or soy powder, is a healthy low-fat, high-protein, appetite satisfying snack.

10. *Sugar-free Jell-O®* or sugar free pudding, topped with fat-free whipped cream. is a tasty, sweet-tooth satisfying snack.

EATING WHEN AWAY FROM HOME:

1. When eating out, choose low-fat foods without sauces, like broiled fish or chicken with a large tossed salad. Avoid alcohol, since it can increase your appetite, and add extra calories. If you like a drink with dinner, a wine spritzer is a good substitute, which is relatively low in total calorie value. Red wine (4 oz.) or a light beer every other night is also acceptable.

2. Don't be afraid to send back your meal in a restaurant if they didn't follow your order instructions. If you asked for steamed vegetables, baked potato, and broiled fish without butter, that's the way it should arrive on your plate.

3. At weddings and other parties choose the fresh vegetables and fruits without the dips. Avoid those fat-laden little appetizers with toothpicks in them. Consider the toothpicks red warning flags to stay away!

4. When traveling by air, order ahead for a low-fat meal when making reservations. They're available! Otherwise, if it is a short flight, have a low-fat snack prior to boarding.

5. Italian: Spaghetti or linguini is lower in fat than wider pastas that are often made with eggs. Try to order (when dining out) or buy whole grain pasta or spinach noodles for their high-fiber content. Stick to tomato or marinara sauces (however, some have too much oil, and you can have the waiter drain the oil from the pasta and bring back your dish). Seafood-based sauces without cream are also good substitutes.

6. Pizza can be ordered without cheese (tomato pie) and then add on a variety of fresh vegetables. If you want cheese, sprinkle on a little Parmesan cheese. Always blot off the extra fat on top of the pizza with a paper towel or napkin to absorb fat. By using this tip you can remove more than 50% of the additional fat calories from the pizza.

7. Chinese restaurants: Stir-fry foods are better than deep-fried. Choose dishes with grains and vegetables. Order brown rice instead of white rice for the extra fiber content (not fried rice, which also comes out brown in color but is low in fiber). Ask to have your food prepared without soy sauce or MSG. Choose vegetable wonton soup or any vegetable-based soup rather than meat-based soups.

8. Mexican foods are great, if you can stay away from the deep-fried tortilla chips and order oven-baked chips with salsa instead. Skip the sour cream and guacamole (avocado), both of which are high in fat. Soft corn tortillas (tostadas or enchiladas) with chicken, tomato sauce and onions are good low-fat choices. Burritos or fajitas without sour cream or guacamole are excellent choices with lettuce, tomato and onion, and can be considered low-fat dishes. Avoid regular refried beans, deep-fried chimichangas, beef taco salad and deep-fried tortilla chips.

9. If you find that you have to eat at a fast food restaurant, order a junior or children's hamburger without the cheese. Skip the fries and add a diet soda or unsweetened iced tea to your sandwich.

10. Make sure you drink a bottle of water before and during your meal.

CALORIES DON'T COUNT—YES THEY DO!

According to a recent study in the *Journal of the American Medical Association,* there is a no magic formula to losing weight. You can lose weight by following a variety of different diet programs; however, the one thing that always counts is the number of calories that you consume vs. the number of calories that you burn daily.

Yes, even those horrendous, low-carbohydrate diets work, but that's because they restrict calories also, not just carbohydrates. Also, they work because you are creating an unhealthy condition found in diabetics called ketosis, where you are burning protein instead of fat to lose weight. Unfortunately, the weight comes back twice as fast when you stop the diet, if you are fortunate enough not to have damaged your liver or kidneys while you were on this unhealthy diet.

Unfortunately, Americans have been gaining so much weight in the last twenty years that obesity is becoming an actual epidemic. Over 60% of adults are overweight, which includes approximately 30% who are considered obese. This trend has almost tripled in teenagers during this same time period. After reviewing over one hundred diet studies over a period of 10 years since 2000, the researchers concluded that if you want to lose weight, you should consume fewer calories daily over a long period of time.

A low-fat, high-fiber diet with moderate amounts of protein, is the single, best weight loss diet that you can follow for good health and permanent weight loss. It's called the *Diet Fit-Step Plan*. There are no dangerous side effects, no feelings of hunger, and along with permanent weight loss, you have the added benefit of a diet that is actually good for you. You will lose weight, and lower your incidence of heart disease, hypertension, strokes, dementia, and several forms of cancer. This diet, by its very nature, turns out to be a low-calorie diet in disguise, and what's more, it actually works and keeps on working.

Food Journal

It is important to keep track of when and what you eat at each and every meal, including snacks. It is just as important to be conscious of why you eat, especially when you are nibbling snacks unconsciously throughout the day, or eating more calories than you should consume at meal time. For example, when you are watching TV and not paying attention to what you were eating. Were you in a meeting or at work or talking on the phone and eating junk food without really noticing what you were eating at the time? A food journal can help you solve these problem areas by keeping an accurate record of what you actually eat at each and every meal on each and every day. This record will enable you to establish a more realistic diet plan as you move forward on your Diet Fit-Step weight loss plan.

You can keep your record of your food diary in a notebook or you can do it online. A food journal gives you a basic guideline of what you have been doing wrong and the means to correct your food eating habits. Make sure that you record everything that you consumed in any given 24 hour period. A food journal can help you solve these problem areas by keeping an accurate record of what you actually eat at each and every meal, on each and every day. It's probably easier and more efficient to just record the number of grams of fat, no more than 35 grams a day, and also record the number of grams of fiber, no less than 35 grams per day. This record will enable you to establish a more realistic diet plan as you move forward on your Diet Fit-Step weight loss plan.

Why Women Gain Weight Easily

- Unfortunately, women gain weight easier and faster than men, which is partially due to a woman's slower metabolism. Men have more muscle mass and burn fat at a faster rate than women. So it is important that women exercise regularly in order to burn calories and to increase their metabolic rates. Women, however, have a distinct advantage over men in that they naturally have more sustained endurance when they exercise. So that women who engage in a regular sustained aerobic exercise program burn more fat calories than men who do strenuous exercises for short periods of time, since quick bursts of energy burn primarily carbohydrates rather than fat. Therefore, sustained aerobic exercise helps women increase their metabolic rates during exercise and also at rest.

- It also takes longer for a woman to digest food than it does for a man. Because of the slower production of certain digestive enzymes, women metabolize fat and a number of medications including alcohol at a slower rate than men. Fat in a woman's diet therefore causes her to gain weight easily because of this inability to digest and metabolize fat quickly.

- So it's no wonder that fat in a woman's diet is just about the worst thing that she can have in order to lose weight and stay healthy. Fat contains 9 calories per gram, and combined with a women's slower rate of metabolism, considerably more fat is stored in her fat cells.

- Increasing lean protein and high-fiber complex carbohydrates into a woman's diet and reducing saturated fats makes it much easier for her to digest and absorb food for the maximum weight-loss effect.

- Low carbohydrate diets, which are essentially high fat diets, make it even more difficult for women to lose weight, and, in particular, to keep the weight off. These diets don't work and they are very toxic to your body. Initial weight loss is always followed by marked rebound weight gain.

Portion Control

Portion control is the key to any successful diet. Serve your meals on small plates to limit the amount that you eat. Eat slowly and stop when you feel full, no matter how much food is left on the plate. Remember that you don't have to finish everything on your plate. Remember, in order to lose weight, you must eat less food. People have a tendency to clean their plates, no matter how large the portion size is. Avoid oversized bowls and plates at home, which tend to hold larger portions. Concentrate on smaller servings and pause during a meal to give your appetite control mechanism time to let you know that you're actually full, and be careful not to eat fast, because you will consume mass quantities of calories before you'll ever know that you're not hungry any longer.

1. Drink one cup of fat-free milk instead of one cup of whole milk. Add nonfat milk to your coffee, cappuccino, or lattes.

2. Use 1 tablespoon of mustard, ketchup, or fat-free mayonnaise instead of regular mayonnaise in salads or on sandwiches. Mix ketchup and nonfat mayonnaise to make a delicious Russian dressing. Served on a wedge of iceberg lettuce, it makes a tasty snack.

3. Share a small bag of potato chips or French fries with a friend, or skip them altogether, or just taste three or four and throw the bag away.

4. Cut a slice of pizza in half and save the other half for later in the day. Also, blot the pizza with a few napkins to absorb the extra fat and calories

5. Check serving sizes of your favorite foods when you eat out. For example:
    a. One-half cup of cooked cereal or pasta at home is equivalent to a single serving size; however, restaurant portions are equivalent to approximately three serving sizes, and that's before they even add the sauce.

b. One-half of a bagel is one serving, but a deli bagel is equivalent to at least 2½ servings.

c. One small pancake or waffle at home is equal to one serving size, but in a restaurant, one pancake is about two and one-half servings.

d. A dozen potato chips or tortilla chips equal approximately one serving; however, a small bag contains at least two to three servings.

6. Always check the serving sizes on any prepackaged food that you get. You will be surprised that some of them say that the contents contain two or three serving sizes. Most people, when they consume a package of processed foods, assume that it is one serving size, when, in actuality, it may be two to three serving sizes.

7. If you're eating at home, use small plates, and when you feel full take your plate into the kitchen and return to the table. If there is no plate at the table then there is no more food to pick at.

8. Always check the labels when buying food. Make sure that the saturated fat and the sugar contents are low. The first listed ingredient on the ingredients label is the one that contains the highest concentration in the food that you are buying. If sugars or fats are listed first, then put it back on the shelf.

Dr. Walk's Fast Food Tips

Most fast foods are so high in calories, saturated fats, and sodium that they not only make us fatter, but they also cause the build-up of fat in our arteries, which can eventually cause heart attacks, strokes, and high blood pressure. Sometimes when you're traveling, fast-food restaurants are your only choices. It's often very difficult to make good choices from these fast-food restaurants; however, it's not impossible if you use common sense and a lot of will power.

The Worst Fast Foods

1. The average double cheeseburger, with large fries and a large soda, contains approximately 1,800-2,000 calories, and approximately 100 grams of fat, of which almost 40 grams are saturated fat. It also contains approximately 1,500 mg of sodium. So, for most people, that amounts to the number of calories that they would consume in one day and three to four times the amount of fat and salt that they would consume in any given day.

2. Two slices of pizza with extra cheese and/or meat contain 750-800 calories, 35-40 grams of fat (15 grams of saturated fat), and 2,000 mg of sodium.

3. Fried fish sandwiches contain approximately 900 calories, 40 grams of fat (15 grams saturated fat), and 1,200 mg of sodium.

4. Nachos with cheese and sour cream contain 1,200-1,300 calories, 80 grams of fat (25 grams saturated fat), and 2,500 mg of salt.

5. A chocolate milkshake contains almost 800 calories and 40 grams of fat, of which 25 grams are saturated.

6. A large coke contains 200 calories.

7. Large fries contain 600+ calories, 20 grams of fat, and 10-12 grams of saturated fat and 1,500 mg of salt.

8. Fried chicken or a fried chicken wrap with cheese and sauce contains 700 calories and 44 grams of fat (12 grams of saturated fat), and 2,000 mg of salt.

THE BEST FAST FOODS

1. Choose a single hamburger without cheese or sauce. Add lettuce, tomato, and onion, with or without ketchup or nonfat mayo, and skip the fries and order a diet soda.

2. Order a grilled chicken sandwich without the mayo or better yet, a grilled chicken Caesar salad with fat-free herb vinaigrette dressing.

3. A good choice is a small vegetable chili without cheese.

4. Soft chicken taco without sauce.

5. Order a large salad plain, or add grilled chicken, and add fat-free dressing.

6. Sliced roast beef sandwich without the sauce.

7. If you must have fries, order the smallest bag and either split with a friend or toss in the trash when you've finished less than one-half.

8. Baked potato chips (small bag) without hydrogenated oils or trans-fats are low in saturated fats and calories.

9. Pizza is a great fast food. According to *Harvard School of Public Health*, tomato sauce contains an antioxidant called *lycopene*, which has been proven to reduce the risk of heart disease and certain forms of cancer, including breast and prostate cancer. A study of over 5,000 people showed that those who ate pizza one to two times per week decreased their risk of different forms of cancer by over 50%. This antioxidant also is a blood pressure and cholesterol lowering agent. Tomato sauce has more lycopene than just ordinary tomatoes, since it is thought to be the heating process of tomatoes that releases the healthy lycopene into the tomato sauce.

    Pizza is also more filling than many foods, causing you to eat fewer calories and become appetite-satisfied earlier. You can bump up the lycopene content and decrease the calorie content of pizza by ordering your pizza with light cheese, and extra tomato sauce.

Or you can order a tomato pie or pizza without cheese. If you do order a regular pizza; make sure you use several napkins to blot up the extra fat before eating. You can reduce the total calorie content of each piece of pizza by more than 25% by using this fat-blotting napkin method. Although pizza, in general, has a lot of calories, there are ways to make it a healthful, low calorie food. Adding lots of veggies to a slice of pizza increases its health benefits, providing you stay away from unhealthy toppings like pepperoni and sausage. So, all in all, a slice of pizza can be a healthy, low-fat food to add to your diet, provided you follow the above guidelines.

10. A soft pretzel is an excellent appetite-satisfying, low-fat snack. The best soft pretzels are those labeled SUPERPRETZEL®. These soft pretzels are sold in most foods and convenience stores, fast-food restaurants, and sports stadiums. They are also found in the frozen-food section of your supermarket or grocery store. These pretzels contain 34 grams carbohydrate, 1 gram of fiber; and 5 grams of protein. They are also extremely low in fat (1 gram of total fat and zero grams of cholesterol, saturated fats and trans-fats).Without added salt, these pretzels contain only 130mg. of sodium. This soft pretzel is very filling, and even if you only eat a portion of it, your hunger mechanism will be promptly satisfied. A favorite way to enjoy a SUPERPRETZEL® is with mustard, to enhance its flavor.

BEWARE RESTAURANT DINING

Recently, research shows that you eat more when you are dining with more people. This is especially true if the people you are eating with consume larger amounts of food. Your appetite goes into overdrive when you are with several people, especially if you are talking and enjoying yourself with friends. What happens is that with the excitement of dining with friends, your appetite mechanism doesn't shut off easily, since you're talking and having fun. Before you know it, you're eating much more than you should have eaten, while not realizing the total amount of food that you consumed.

Plan in advance if you're going to have dinner with friends. Order a low-fat, low-calorie meal, regardless of what your dinner companions order. Concentrate on taking small bites and eating slowly while eating with friends. Also, stop your meal while talking, so that you're not consuming mass quantities of food without realizing this fact. If you're a woman dining with a man, you should know that men can eat much more food than you can without gaining weight. Who said life was fair! Men burn more calories quickly because of testosterone that builds muscle mass, which causes their metabolism to run faster. So men can actually eat more calories than women do without gaining weight easily. Here are some tips that you should use to eat less when you're dining with friends or family:

1. Chew your food slowly. Put your fork down between bites.

2. Stop eating when talking and resume eating slowly when conversation stops.

3. Don't be afraid to leave food on your plate.

4. Never order a meal to coincide with what your friends are ordering. Fatty, high-calorie meals sound good when someone else orders them; however, don't let their order be contagious.

5. Don't try to keep up the pace with a fast eater at your table. They probably have no idea what or how much they are eating. Be careful of alcoholic beverages when dining with friends. Never order more than one drink if you do drink. If you're not a drinker, don't be afraid to not order a drink. Just get water or club soda with a twist. If you'd like a light drink, however, get a white wine spritzer (half the wine, half the calories, and club soda).

6. When dining in a restaurant, it's a good idea to ask the waiter to wrap half of your meal before or after they bring it to the table. Since restaurant meals are usually considerably larger (two to three times as large) than you serve at home, you'll have enough left-over for a second meal the next day.

7. Most restaurant dishes seem to have to add high-fat sauces and dressings to everything from meats to salads. Always request the sauce or dressing on the side and don't be afraid to leave half the dinner on your plate (or take it home for another meal).

8. At a restaurant, if you can split a meal with a friend or relative, try to do so, even if there's a sharing charge. Also split a dessert with your companion to enjoy the sweet taste without eating extra calories.

9. Don't be tempted by your dining companions to order similar foods or drinks, especially if they fall outside the parameters of the Diet-Step: 35/35 weight-loss plan.

10. The increase in obesity seems to coincide with the meals eaten out at restaurants, and not just fast-food restaurants. The portion sizes in restaurants are huge compared to the amount that you eat at home. Always choose grilled or baked foods without breading. Order hardy vegetable soup whenever possible and avoid cream soups. And, most importantly, don't finish those oversized meals that most restaurants put in front of you, or you can order two appetizers instead of one large

entrée. Also remember that when you're dining with friends or relatives, you're not obligated to keep up with the amount of food and drinks that they are consuming. Eat at your own pace and when you feel full, stop eating and wait until your companions are finished. Remember, dining is not a contest as to who can eat and drink the most.

METABOLIC MYSTERY

Protein is the essential building block for the maintenance and repair of the body's cells, tissues, and organs. Protein is the fuel that keeps your metabolic engine working efficiently. An adequate protein intake controls and regulates your body's metabolism and also regulates your blood sugar and insulin levels. Protein therefore is essential not only for good health, but it has the ability to control your body's appetite (the appestat), which keeps your hunger satisfied. Small to moderate amounts of protein eaten with every meal help you to lose weight by controlling your appetite and by burning more fat calories. Protein also regulates the metabolism of both fat and carbohydrate in your body. Protein is the metabolic wizard that controls your metabolism, builds muscle, burns fat, and helps you to lose weight in a safe and healthy manner.

Recent research has also shown that protein can protect older people from hip fractures, because protein builds bone density and increases muscle strength from the legs that support the hip joints. People who ate the least amount of protein suffered 50% more hip fractures than those who ate the most amount of protein.

PROTEIN DIET CLUES

HEALTHY PROTEIN

It is important to add lean, healthy protein to your diet in the form of very lean meat, fish and poultry without skin; nonfat milk and low-fat cheeses, including yogurt; and vegetable protein, including tofu, beans, nuts and legumes. When you are on a low calorie diet, your body needs more protein for the production of energy and your body's cell maintenance. Avoid unhealthy, high animal fat proteins, such as cheeseburgers, hotdogs, sausage, bacon, butter and margarine.

Protein is the essential nutrient responsible for the maintenance and repair of all your organs, tissues, muscles, brain and bones. All foods are sources of energy; however, protein provides a greater boost in energy levels since it is absorbed slowly and thus produces a constant source of energy.

HEALTHY PROTEIN MEALS

Balance your meals by adding a small amount of lean protein to each meal:

1. Hard-boiled egg on a slice of whole wheat bread or English muffin.

2. Tuna melt with low-fat cheese on whole wheat bread with tomato slice.

3. Small Caesar salad with Romaine lettuce, low-fat Parmesan cheese and an ounce of grilled chicken and low-fat Caesar dressing on the side.

4. One slice of whole wheat bread with a poached egg.

5. A cup of cooked oatmeal or high-protein cold cereal with cinnamon and ¼ cup of raisons and non-fat milk.

6. A fried egg with nonfat spray and a slice of whole wheat bread.

7. A veggie burger on whole wheat bread or bun with lettuce, tomato, onion and ketchup or a ½ veggie hoagie on scooped-out Italian roll.

8. A soft corn tortilla with fat free refried beans, shredded low-fat cheese, lettuce, tomato and salsa.

9. A slice of pizza topped with veggies and a side salad with non fat dressing on side.

10. 2 ounces lean roast beef with horseradish and small baked potato or yam with skin, 1 cup steamed veggies and small whole wheat roll.

11. One cup of whole wheat spaghetti with 12 clams or mussels, garlic, ⅓ cup white wine, ¾ tsp. olive oil, and large tossed salad.

12. One cup of low-fat macaroni and cheese with a cup of zucchini, diced tomatoes, onions and garlic, and a small sweet potato and steamed fresh carrots.

13. Nuts, particularly walnuts and almonds, are rich in monounsaturated fats, and cause the brain to release a hormone which actually shuts down the appetite control mechanism in the brain and prevents hunger. Nuts are also packed with protein and help reduce the risk of heart disease.

14. Turkey breast or white meat of chicken breast on whole wheat with lettuce, tomato and non-fat mayonnaise.

15. Any grilled or poached fresh fish is high in protein.

16. Grilled low-fat cheese on whole wheat bread with tomato.

17. Egg white omlette with veggies.

18. Eggs also are a good source of healthy protein and are especially rich in heart and brain healthy omega-3 fatty acids. Previously, eggs were thought to be unhealthy because of their high concentration of cholesterol. Recent studies however,

have proven otherwise. In an eight year study of more than 125,000 men and women, there appeared to be no link shown between the consumption of eggs and the risks of stroke or coronary heart disease, except among those people with diabetes. It is interesting to note that women who ate more than one egg per day had the lowest risk of coronary heart disease. Eggs are very low in saturated fats and contain many healthy ingredients like lutein and xanthein which help to keep your eyes from developing cataracts and macular degeneration. It's still a good idea to limit your intake of eggs to one egg three or four times a week, and substitute egg whites the rest of the week.

Harmful Protein

Most low carbohydrate, high-fat, animal protein diets have you eating 3-4 times more protein than the recommended dietary allowance, and in most cases, the high-protein you are actually eating is the harmful, high fat kind. These diets tax your kidneys and leach out calcium from your bones, in addition to contributing to elevated blood cholesterol which leads to heart disease and strokes. Minimize all fatty meats (primarily beef, and liver, pork, lamb, ham, sausage, bacon, scrapple, hot dogs, and lunch-meats). Limit fatty fowl like duck, dark meat of chicken and turkey and chicken and turkey skin. Also eliminate whole milk and whole milk dairy products, butter, margarine, solid fat spreads, saturated oils, and limit your intake of most polyunsaturated oils.

BEAT FOOD CRAVINGS

People who are anxious or stressed out have a tendency to crave sweets and high-calorie foods. Anxiety and stress cause your adrenal glands and pituitary gland to produce certain hormones that stimulate your brain's hunger mechanism to crave refined sugars and carbohydrates (cakes, pies, doughnuts, and candy bars). These quick-fix carbs tend to quell anxiety temporarily by the sudden rise in blood sugar, which causes a feeling of calm. However, a rapid rise in blood sugar causes a rapid spike in insulin which causes a more rapid drop in blood sugar.

You can beat anxiety and stress food cravings by eating low-calorie, crunchy foods, such as apples, celery, carrot sticks, or low-fat pretzels (whole-wheat or sourdough). The crunch factor gives your stress-induced anxiety time to cool down without causing a rapid rise in your blood sugar. The actual process of chewing causes your facial and neck muscles to relax, which, in turn, relieves stress and tension.

If you are depressed or sad, your first inclination is also to head for the sweet bar instead of the salad bar. The quick-fix of sugar raises the blood sugar, which, in turn, spikes the pancreas's insulin production. High levels of insulin in the blood increase the production of *serotonin*, which improves your emotional mood. You feel more relaxed and mellow, which is actually how antidepressant drugs work, by increasing your brain's serotonin levels. Unfortunately, serotonin levels plummet after insulin levels drop, and the feeling of sadness and depression quickly returns. To combat this feeling, you can boost your serotonin levels for longer periods of time by eating fruits when you are feeling down. Fruits only gradually increase the level of blood sugar because fruit sugar, or fructose, is slowly absorbed. Insulin levels then become graduated, causing a sustained, long-lived blood and brain serotonin levels.

People who eat because they are bored or just plain tired often eat high-calorie, refined sugar carbohydrate snacks, like cakes and candies, which are readily available and easy to buy or consume.

A mocha caffeinated latte may taste good, but the caffeine and sugar interfere with the production of endorphins and serotonin. Instead of feeling relaxed and calm, you will feel edgy and wired. Nuts, particularly almonds and walnuts, are great boredom snacks, since they provide omega-3 fatty acids that can relieve the feelings of fatigue and boredom. Combined with raisins, nuts make the ideal feel-good, energy-boosting snack.

THE MYSTERY OF THE SCALE

Remember, no one loses weight in a straight line. When you are on a diet, you initially lose weight, and then your weight loss levels off. This occurs even though you are eating exactly the same amount as you were when you lost the initial weight. This leveling-off period or *plateau* is the single most hazardous part of any diet program. The reason is that once you've reach the diet plateau, you begin to become discouraged, and you'll say, "I'm still on the same diet, but I haven't lost a pound in over a week." Discouragement leads to frustration, and next you'll say, "The heck with the diet. I may as well enjoy myself and eat something I really like, since I haven't lost weight anyway." At this point, 90 percent of all diets are doomed to failure, since the weight loss pattern now reverses itself and becomes a *weight gain pattern*.

If you can stick out this plateau period, which incidentally is *always temporary*, you'll be surprised to see that the weight loss begins to pick up speed again. It may take a week or two, at the most, but if you are patient, you will again start to lose those unwanted pounds. No one has ever satisfactorily explained this plateau period; however, physiologists believe that it is probably due to *a temporary readjustment of the body's metabolism* in response to the initial weight loss. No matter what the reason is, however, you will always break through the plateau period, providing you don't become discouraged or frustrated. Weight loss will again resume its downward progress toward your ideal weight goal.

This plateau period is one of the main reasons that I insist that my patients do not weigh themselves daily. In fact, **weighing yourself every day is hazardous to your diet**. The reason for this is twofold. First, when you weigh yourself daily and see that you are losing weight, you become happy and elated, and subconsciously you will eat to celebrate. Secondly, if you see that you are not losing weight as fast as you "think" you should, you become depressed and anxious, and sometime during that day you will subconsciously eat because of frustration. So, the rule of thumb is: **The more you weigh yourself, the more you eat!** Believe me, it is true. I've seen my patients go through this frustrating daily weighing process thousands of times. No one on a diet should weigh themselves more than once a week, and then you will get a true measure of the effectiveness of your diet. If you must weigh yourself, then Wednesday is the best day to weigh yourself each week. Monday and Friday are the worst days for weighing in, since they follow and precede the weekend and lead to frustrating eating binges. It took a long time to gain all that weight; you can't take it off overnight. Be patient and you'll take off those unwanted pounds in record time.

The Case of the Unwanted Pounds

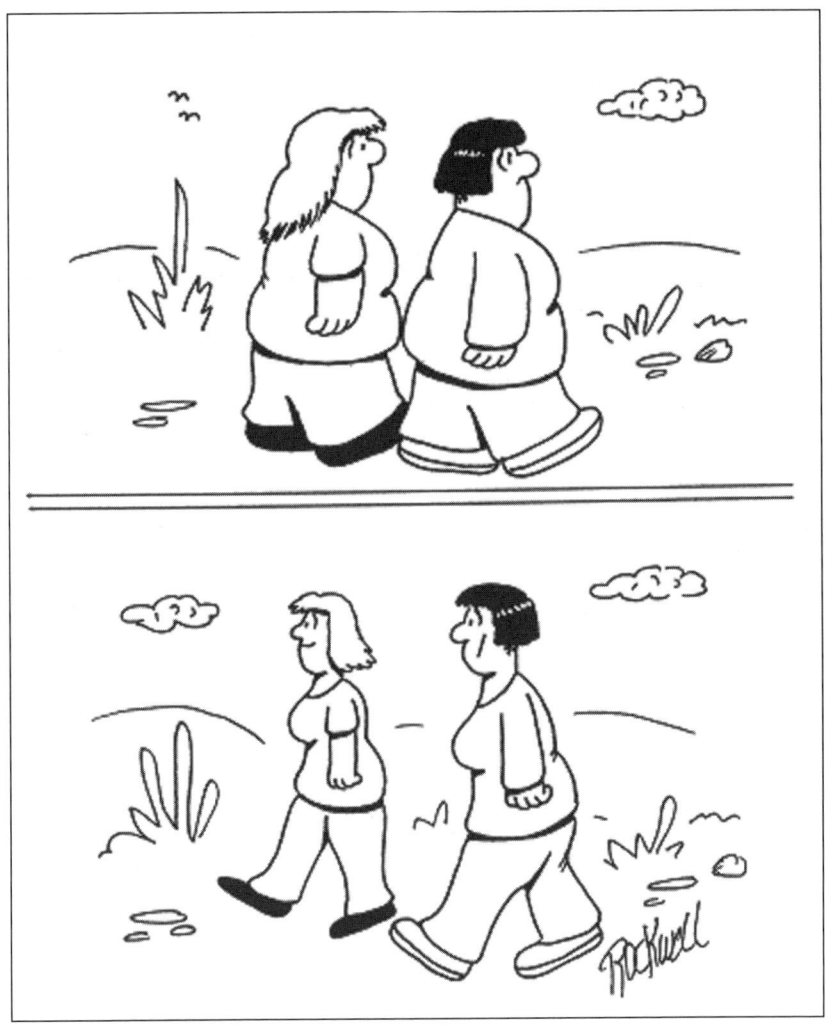

"I don't know about you, but I feel thinner already—and we've only been walking for 35 minutes!"

6

Get Fit & Trim in 35 Minutes

The 2nd component of the Diet Fit-Step Mystery Plan is the *Fit-Step: 35 minute six day per week aerobic walking plan.* The walking component of the Fit Step Plan is the process that causes your body's metabolism to burn calories during and also after you're walking. You'll be surprised how good you feel after your 35 minute walk, with increased energy and vigor. The additional flow of oxygen throughout your bloodstream will increase your metabolic rate, so that you will burn calories more quickly. This increase in metabolism will allow you to lose weight more quickly and will improve your cardiovascular fitness.

With the advent of the computer age, people are forced by design to do less and less physical labor. It would seem logical that this would result in more energy being available for other activities. However, how many times have you noticed that the less you do, the more tired you feel, whereas the more active you are, the more energy you have for other activities? Exercise improves the efficiency of the lungs, the heart and the circulatory system in their ability to take in and deliver oxygen throughout the entire body.

This oxygen is the catalyst which burns the fuel (food) we take in to produce energy. Consequently, the more oxygen we take in, the more energy we have for all of our activities. Oxygen is the vital ingredient that is necessary for our survival. Since oxygen can't be stored, our cells need a continuous supply in order to remain healthy. Walking increases your body's ability to extract oxygen from the air, so that increased amounts of oxygen are available for every organ, tissue and cell in the body. So let's take that first step for energy, fitness and pep. Walking six days per week will keep a fresh supply of oxygen flowing through your blood vessels to all of your body's cells. A Fit-Step® a day keeps the doctor away.

LOSE WEIGHT WITH THE FIT STEP®

Thirty-five minutes walking briskly (approximately 3.5 mph) every day except Sunday is all that you need to do in the Fit-Step Plan. Either 35 minutes outdoors (walking) or 35 minutes indoors (stationary bike or treadmill) will provide you with maximum cardiovascular fitness, good health, and boundless energy. Remember, this 35 minute walk is a basic part of your weight loss program on the Fit-Step® Plan. Your 35 minute walk, 6 days per week, is what burns the extra calories needed to lose additional weight and to decrease your appetite. The Fit-Step® walking plan also provides the fuel that powers your energy level throughout your day. *When you combine the Fit-Step Plan with the Diet-Step Plan, you have the added power to burn additional calories on the Diet Fit-Step Mystery Plan.*

When you first start your Fit-Step walking program, pick a level terrain, since hills place too much strain and stress on your legs, hips and back muscles. Concentrate on maintaining erect posture while walking. Walk with your shoulders relaxed and your arms carried in a relatively low position with natural motion at the elbow. Don't hold your arms too high when you walk, otherwise you will develop muscle spasms and pain in your neck, back and shoulder muscles.

Make sure you walk at a brisk pace (approximately 3½ mph) for maximum efficiency. When you begin walking, your respiration and heart rate will automatically become faster; however, if you feel short of breath or tired, then you're probably walking too fast. Remember to stop whenever you are tired or fatigued and then resume walking after resting. Concentrate on walking naturally, putting energy into each step. Soon you will begin to feel relaxed and comfortable as your stride becomes smooth and effortless. Walk with an even steady gait and your own rhythm of walking will automatically develop into an unconscious synchronous movement.

ONLY 21 DAYS TO REACH YOUR PEAK

Your Fit-Step walking program should be planned to meet your individual schedule; however, when you begin it's a good idea to walk at a specific time every day to ensure regularity and consistency. You will be able to vary your schedule once you have started the program. Lunchtime, for example, is an ideal time to plan a 35 minute walk since it combines both calorie burning and calorie reduction. If you have less time for lunch, you'll eat less.

Most people can start their daily walking exercise for 35 minutes at a time, six days per week. If you're really out of shape, then you can gradually build up to your 6 day per week, 35 minute walking plan. The first week, walk 10 minutes a day, six days per week. The second week, walk 20 minutes a day, six days per week, and the third week walk 30 minutes, 6 days per week. After the first 21 days, you're ready for your regular 35 minute walk six days per week.

Remember, the speed of walking is not important, unless you are walking too slowly (under 2 mph). A brisk walking speed of 3.5 miles per hour is a good walking speed for maximum calorie burning and aerobic physical fitness. The most important factor is that you walk regularly at a relatively brisk pace. If you become tired easily, get short of breath, develop pain anywhere or if any other unusual symptoms occur, check with your physician immediately.

THE EXERCISE FALLACIES

Why are there so many exercise dropouts? And why don't many men and women even try to begin an exercise plan in the first place? Most people think that an exercise program is futile, since they'll never be able to look like the perfect bodies in the magazines or at the gym. You don't have to be put into a situation where you feel intimidated by an instructor in a gym or on an exercise video.

Most people think physical fitness is actually harder than it is. And they feel that exercise programs are too complicated, when they hear terms like "oxygen consumption," "body fat composition," "body mass index," "lean muscle mass," etc. It all sounds too complicated and too boring for most men and women to begin exercising in any formalized program.

What most people don't realize is that they don't have to participate in a regimented exercise program to see results. They don't have to join a gym or health club and be intimidated by a twenty-year-old fitness instructor with boundless energy. And they don't have to exercise vigorously or do strenuous exercises in order to obtain maximum fitness and to develop a lean, trim body. As we've already discussed, exercise doesn't have to be strenuous to be beneficial. Also, exercise doesn't have to be painful in order to be gainful. Exercise can really be fun! It can be easy to follow and easy to continue. It doesn't have to be boring or a drudgery that has to be done. That's why the Fit-Step Plan was devised—in order to make it easy for people to become fit and trim, and to make it easy for them to maintain their new level of fitness.

There are two main fallacies about exercising that you should be aware of. The first is the **"No Pain – No Gain"** myth which is completely false. An exercise doesn't have to be painful to be beneficial. In fact the reverse is actually true in that moderate exercise is more beneficial and less hazardous than strenuous exercises.

The second fallacy is the **"Target Heart Rate Zone"** myth. No one has ever proved that you have to get your heart rate up to astronomical numbers to insure cardiovascular fitness. Here in fact, the reverse is also true, in that moderate exercise provides better cardiovascular fitness than strenuous exercise. Both of these so-called exercise precepts are what makes many men and women discontinue their exercise plans or never start them in the first place. Once you realize that both of these so-called concepts are fallacies or myths and that it is not necessary to make exercise painful or stressful, you can begin to begin to relax and enjoy the **Fit-Step Plan.**

OTHER COMMON EXERCISE MYTHS:

1. If you're exercising strenuously, and you're breathing rapidly and shallowly during your exercise, then you're not delivering enough oxygen into the lungs, where it can be absorbed into the bloodstream. If however, you walk at a moderately brisk pace, and take longer deeper breaths while exercising, you're able to deliver more oxygen deep into your lung tissues, and thus absorb more oxygen into your bloodstream.

2. Be careful when increasing your walking speed, and resist the temptation to stretch your stride too far. If you stretch your stride too far, then you will throw off your balance while walking, and put extra stress on your knees and shin bones.

3. There is no such thing as "*spot reduction*" while doing different exercises. For instance, you won't remove fat deposits in your buttocks on a stair climber or elliptical machine. Also, doing sit-ups won't remove excess fat around your waist. When you follow a healthy low-fat, high fiber diet, combined with a well-rounded exercise program like walking or walking with light hand-held weights, fat will be burned gradually from fat deposits all over your body.

Fit-Step® Mystery Walking Tips

1. Our bodies are one of the few machines that break down when not in use. A physically active person is one who is both physically and mentally alert. A walking program can actually slow down the aging process and add years to our lives. Walking has been proven to be a significant factor in the prevention of heart and vascular disease. It strengthens the heart muscle, improves the lung's efficiency, and lowers the blood pressure by keeping the blood vessels flexible. Walking will add years to your life, and life to your years!

2. In order to walk comfortably and efficiently without tiring, you should balance your body weight over the feet or just slightly ahead of them. Keep your body relaxed, and your knees bent slightly, utilizing a steady, even pace, and a brisk walking stride. To obtain the most benefit out of your walking program you should try to walk with the Fit-Step® heel-and-toe method, pointing your feet straight ahead. By utilizing this method, your leg muscles are used more efficiently, and this results in an overall increased blood supply to the peripheral circulation (in particular the legs and feet) and to the general circulation (all of the body's cells, tissues and organs).

3. The leading leg is brought forward in front of the body, thus enabling the heel of the lead foot to touch the ground just before the ball of the foot and the toes. Your weight is then shifted forward so that when your heel is raised, your toes will push off for the next step. Your arms and shoulders should be relaxed, and they will swing automatically with each stride you take. Before long, you will develop a natural rhythm, pace, and stride as you walk. The Fit-Step® walking method uses the calf muscles to pump the blood up the leg veins back to the heart and lungs, and then out through the arteries to all your body's cells, tissues, and organs. This walking method keeps your body lean and your arteries clean.

4. When you walk, don't slouch. Walk tall! The way to walk is with your head up, shoulders back, stomach in, and your chest out. Learning to walk tall comes with practice, but after a while, this stance will become a natural part of your Fit-Step® walking style. Your stride is the single most important aspect of your walk.

5. There is no correct stride length. Stretch as much as you can without straining when you are walking. Thrust your legs forward briskly, swing your arms vigorously and feel your energy surge forth as you walk with the Fit-Step® stride.

6. Keep your pace steady, never push and don't try to accelerate your speed when walking. If you do get tired after a short period of time, stop and rest and then re-start again at a steady and even pace. Don't rush; just walk at a comfortable Fit-Step pace. Your rhythm of walking is a condition that will come naturally as you continue your walking program. Keep your body relaxed and your stride steady and even, and your rhythm will develop naturally. Uneven walking surfaces that you encounter will control your rhythm, especially going down or uphill. Don't fight it, just walk naturally and you'll be doing the Fit-Step.

7. The Fit-Step walking method is the ideal weight control and fitness program. Studies in human physiology have proven that walking acts as a weight reduction plan without actually dieting and a fitness program without strenuous exercises. Too often today we allow a sedentary lifestyle to dominate our daily living. We sit at our desks all day and in front of the TV set in the evenings. We drive to our destination, no matter how close or how far, instead of doing what's easy, natural and healthful—walking. Most of us would rather spend 20 minutes in our cars waiting at the drive-in window of a bank, rather than getting out and walking the length of the parking lot. Even at work, we opt for the elevator even if it's only for a few floors. At the supermarket or shopping mall most of us would rather drive around the parking lot several times, so that we can get a

parking spot closer to the store. These are all good opportunities to do the Fit-Step, not the car-step. Use your feet, not your wheels, and you'll look great and feel full of pep when you do the Fit-Step.

8. Remember, it's the amount of *time* that you walk every day that is more important than the distance or even the speed. If you walk for 35 minutes, six days per week at a brisk pace (approximately 3½ miles per hour), you will burn calories, lose weight, and develop cardiovascular fitness.

Boost Your Energy Level

Once you've started walking for 35 minutes, six days per week, you will begin to notice the many changes brought about by your improved aerobic fitness and maximum oxygen capacity (the uptake and distribution of oxygen through your body). You will have lots of pep and energy, a trim figure, improved breathing capacity and muscle tone, improved exercise tolerance, a better night's sleep, a feeling of peace and relaxation, and a lessening of tension. Once you have completed this 21-day conditioning program, you will have taken the first steps towards improved cardiovascular fitness, good health and a long, happy life. Then all you need to do is *walk 35 minutes every day except Sunday (or any free day of the week) to reap all of the fitness and calorie burning benefits of the Fit-Step Plan.*

The great part about walking as an exercise is that you aren't limited to a particular time or location. Walking doesn't require special clothes or equipment. You can walk before or after work, or if you drive to work, you can park your car a block or two from the office, and walk the rest of the way. If you take the bus or train, get off a stop before your station and walk. An enclosed mall could be the perfect place for your walk in bad weather. Remember to take 35 minutes from your lunch break and walk. Just think of how good that fresh air will feel and smell. Each city or town usually has a guidebook containing historical sites, restaurants, shops of interest, cultural centers and interesting walking paths or tours.

If you live near a park, the country or the seashore, a walking trip will be a refreshing change. Take the time to walk everywhere. Each new area has its own natural beauty. The wonderful world of walking is literally at your feet. Just take that next step for vigor, vim and pep.

INDOOR DIET FIT-STEP® PLAN

It's not necessary to wait until the "weather is better" to go out and walk. There's no excuse for not exercising at home on any day when the weather is inclement. Also take precautions against exercising when it's very hot or humid outdoors. Heat exhaustion and occasionally heat stroke are complications frequently found in those fanatical runners that you see running on hot, humid days. Remember, it's not necessary to walk outdoors if the weather is extremely cold, windy, wet, hot or humid. Here are various indoor exercise alternatives to help you stay on your Fit-Step Plan.

1. STATIONARY FIT-STEP:

This is a combination of walking and running in place. Walk in place for 5 minutes lifting your foot approximately 4 inches off the floor and taking approximately 60 steps a minute (count only when right foot hits floor). Alternate this with 5 minutes of running in place lifting your foot approximately 8 inches off the floor and taking approximately 90 steps a minute (again only count when the right foot hits the floor). Use a padded exercise mat or a thick rug. Wear a padded sneaker or walking shoe. Bare feet will cause foot and leg injuries. Repeat this walk-run cycle twice daily, for a total of 35 minutes. If you tire easily, stop and rest.

2. DANCE FIT-STEP:

Turn on the music and dance for 35 minutes to your favorite music, whether it's pop, jazz, classical, R&B, or any music with a moderately fast beat. Make up your own moves and dance to the beat of the music.

Music can release stress and tension and alleviate anxiety by focusing your thoughts on the music rather than on your problems. Portable CD players or iPods can actually push people to exercise harder. Walking or dancing to music actually helps you to burn more calories and lose more weight while relieving stress and tension.

You can also work out at home to music while on your stationary bike or treadmill. The faster the music, the faster your workout and the more calories you will burn. If you are not into indoor exercise machines then just dance to the music at home. Dancing is a whole body exercise that can be as gentle or as vigorous as you like. Any type of dance step will do. It is your preference whether it is tap, jazz, folk, modern or aerobic dance. You can usually find a video that helps you to dance to your favorite type of dance step.

In a study at Farley Dickinson University it was shown that women who exercise to music, in addition to lowering their calorie intake, lost twice the amount of fat and pounds compared to a group of women who did not listen to music when they exercised. It was thought that the music exercising women were more motivated and pushed themselves harder during their exercise program than those women who did not listen to music while exercising.

3. STATIONARY BIKE FIT-STEP:

One of the easiest ways to continue your indoor Fit-Step program is by using a stationary exercise bicycle. This is the only one-time investment you'll ever need to make as you travel the road towards fitness and good health. No other type of exercise equipment is necessary for your Fit-Step program.

The most important features to look for in a stationary bicycle are a comfortable seat with good support, adjustable handlebars, a chain guard, a quiet pedal and chain, and a solid front wheel. Most come with speedometers to tell the rate that you are pedaling and odometers to tell the mileage that you pedal. An inexpensive stationary bike works just as well as an expensive one. Stationary bikes with moving handlebars are worthless. They claim to exercise the upper half of your body. In reality, they move your arms and back muscles passively, which can result in pulled muscles and strained ligaments.

The stationary bike is the safest and most efficient type of indoor exercise equipment that can be used in place of your outdoor walking program. You can listen to music, watch TV, talk on the telephone, or even read (a bookstand attachment can easily be clamped onto the handle bars) while riding your stationary bike. If the bike comes with a tension dial, leave it on zero or minimal tension. Remember, it is not necessary to strain yourself to develop aerobic fitness. Exercises like walking and the stationary bike can be fun, without being painful or stressful. You may alternate days of outdoor walking and indoor cycling depending on your individual schedule.

You should pedal at a speed of between 10 to 12 miles per hour. If that seems too fast for you, then pedal at a speed that seems comfortable for you. You should begin by dividing your 35 minutes on the bike into two sessions to avoid fatigue, and then very gradually build up to one 35 minute session. Always wear a walking shoe or sneaker (never pedal barefoot or with just socks). A chain guard prevents clothing from getting caught in the bike chain; otherwise roll up your sweats.

4. RECUMBENT STATIONARY BIKES:

Some people feel that their body alignment is more comfortable and natural on a recumbent stationary bike. They also tend to say that the bike seats are more comfortable and ergonomically shaped than seats for upright bikes. Some studies have also shown that the recumbent stationary bike puts less stress on the upper and lower back muscles while pedaling. Recumbent bikes also help to build up the quadriceps muscles more than stationary upright bikes because of the positioning of your legs, and are therefore good for individuals with knee problems. It's an individual choice as to which type of bike feels most comfortable for you. Both bikes provide the same level of aerobic fitness and calorie burning.

5. TREADMILLS:

The treadmill is an effective way to burn calories and build cardiovascular fitness. Manual treadmills are hard on the feet, since you have to push down to make them move and the walking motion is unnatural. Look for motorized treadmills with a deck area (the walking space) with enough length and width to accommodate any stride. The deck area should be at least 18 inches wide by 55 inches long. A cushioned deck is better for your ankles and knees and a thick tread belt is best. You can compare the thickness by the feel when you try out the treadmill or by asking the salesperson for the thickness measurement.

Look for motorized treadmills with a high continuous duty rating of at least 1.5 horsepower as opposed to a motor with a maximum output. Continuous duty motors give you constant maximum power, whereas maximum output motors surge to accommodate short spurts, but you won't be able to walk smoothly for an extended period of time. You can also choose a treadmill with a power incline; however, too much of an incline is bad for the knees and ankles and can put a strain on your back. Also, make sure that the machine has an automatic stop button; if you stumble or feel dizzy, you can push the button and halt the machine instantly. You should begin by dividing your 35 minutes on the treadmill into two sessions to avoid fatigue, and then very gradually build up to one 35 minute session. When you begin to walk on the treadmill, set the speed at 2 miles per hour, and then very gradually build up the speed to 3 or 3.5 miles per hour. If you become fatigued or short of breath, then set the speed to a rate that feels comfortable for you. Remember, it's not a race. Some people find that the treadmill causes knee and/or ankle pain, which results from the constant pounding and impact that the legs sustain. If the treadmill causes recurrent knee or ankle pain, then a recumbent stationary bike or a low-impact elliptical machine may be a better choice for these individuals.

6. ELLIPTICAL FITNESS MACHINES:

This type of machine combines the movement of a treadmill and a stair climber. Your feet loop forward to simulate walking, but the footpads rise and fall with your feet. The elliptical motion provides a no-impact type of exercise, which is great if you have arthritis, knee or back problems that make walking difficult. For maximum exercise, an elliptical machine with dual cross-trainer arms, which move back and forth as you stride, rather than the stationary arms, provides maximum exercise and burns more calories and uses more muscle groups. Most of these machines come with an adjustable ramp incline and resistance settings. However, the normal setting is usually more than adequate for cardiovascular fitness. Also, be careful of small space-saving elliptical machines, since they may not comfortably accommodate a tall person's stride, or may not afford full range of motion. Try out different machines to see which one you're comfortable with. The elliptical machine can be a very good alternative to outdoor walking. You should begin by dividing your 35 minutes on the elliptical machine into two sessions to avoid fatigue, and then very gradually build up to one 35 minute session. If you find that one 35 minute session feels too strenuous or tiring, then just keep up your exercise on this machine divided into two 17½ minute sessions.

7. SWIMMING:

Thirty-five minutes of swimming provides the same aerobic conditioning and cardiovascular fitness benefits as walking and other indoor Fit-Step exercises. Swimming, in fact, has the added benefit of being easy on the joints, especially if you have any form of arthritis or back problems. The reason for this is that swimming puts very little stress on the joints because of the decreased gravity factor provided by the buoyancy of the water. If you have access to an indoor or outdoor swimming pool, then 35 minutes of swimming will fit the bill perfectly for the Fit-Step plan. Water aerobics are excellent non-weight-bearing exercises for fitness, weight-loss, body shaping and for helping to prevent osteoporosis.

8. SKIPPING FIT-STEP:

If you're coordinated enough to use a jump rope, skipping can be a fun indoor exercise. Skip over the rope alternating one foot at a time for 5 minutes and then skip using both feet together for 10 minutes. Use a mat or padded rug with a padded low sneaker or walking shoe. Do this exercise two or three times daily for a total of 35 minutes. If you feel you are not coordinated enough for rope skipping, then skip it!

9. MALL WALKING:

For those of you who don't like to exercise at home when the weather's bad, an indoor mall can be just the place to take your 35 minute walk. Many malls open early before the stores open to accommodate "mall walkers." If you have access to one of these enclosed malls and don't like to stay at home exercising, then by all means, get out there and do the Fit-Step®. Remember to put vigor, vim and pep into your mall walk step. Keep your eyes straight ahead so that you won't be window shopping walking. If you tire easily, then divide your walk into two sessions, totaling 35 minutes.

TRAVEL FIT WITH THE FIT-STEP®

Whether you're taking a vacation or a business trip, you can still keep trim and fit with your walking program. Most major airlines, cruise ships and trains offer special diet menus. If you have to splurge on one meal a day, don't worry. You'll walk it off in no time at all. Cruise ships and trains are ideal for short walks. Walk around the airport concourse while waiting for flights or during layovers. Most major hotels can give you a map of the area for a walking tour. Get up early before your meeting and take a brisk 35 minute walk. Use the stairs whenever possible and walk around the hotel as much as possible if the weather is bad.

Many hotels have small gyms where you can swim or use a stationary bike—take advantage of them if the weather's bad instead of watching TV. Many business trips are associated with a lot of stress and walking can ease away the tension, leaving you more relaxed and more efficient. Speakers always do better after they've had a walk—more brain oxygen and relaxing chemicals (endorphins) and less carbon dioxide result in a sharp, clear, concise speech with no stage jitters. You can keep fit and have lots of energy when you do the Fit-Step. Don't let a little trip, trip you up. Most people feel exhausted after a vacation or a business trip because they sit around all day and stuff their faces with food and drink. Make it a habit to walk at least 35 minutes every day that you're away. You'll return from your travels fit, full of vigor, vim and pep.

MYSTERY DRINK

Most people don't realize that they don't drink enough water. Recent studies have indicated that at least ¾ of adults walk around chronically dehydrated, because they forget for one reason or another to drink the recommended six, 8 oz. glasses of water daily. Chronic dehydration can lead to kidney damage, dizziness, headaches, and irregular heart rhythms, particularly palpitations.

Adequate water consumption is necessary for all the body's metabolic functions and for the health of all of the body's organs, tissues, and cells. Water is essential for digestion, kidney function, respiratory and cardiac health, and the metabolism of the entire body. Without adequate water intake, you run the risk of many health disorders.

One way to keep regularly hydrated is to make sure that you drink water before, during, and after each meal. If you drink just 4 ounces of water at a time frequently throughout the day, you can trick yourself into drinking the recommended six, 8 oz. glasses of water daily. Also, water fills you up without filling you out and helps to decrease your appetite so that you consume fewer calories. Here you have an easy mystery weight loss drink. Dieters who sip water all day tend to lose more weight than people who drink less water daily. Drinking water has a significant effect on a dieter's success, since water has no calories and reduces food cravings which control your appetite by making you feel full with a zero calorie drink.

Surprisingly, water increases the flow of blood to your skin and gives your face a rosy glow by dilating small skin capillaries when you are well-hydrated. Also, good hydration is helpful in providing an increased flow of blood to all of your body's cells which improves your metabolism at a cellular level. Water also helps to prevent kidney stones by diluting substances in the blood like calcium and then flushes these diluted substances out of the body. Urologists suggest that people who have a tendency to develop kidney stones should drink at least six to eight, 8 oz. glasses of water daily. New studies suggest that water also reduces the intensity and duration of migraine headaches. This is apparently due to an increased blood supply to the brain. And lastly, water has been shown to reduce the incidence of colds and flu-like viruses by hydrating the membranes of the nasal and throat passages, making it difficult for viruses to embed themselves in or on dry mucous membranes.

Potassium: Not Just For Runners

Whether your exercise is indoors or outside, if you exercise strenuously, your body can become depleted of both water and potassium. This is the reason that runners are given water and bananas after a sweat-drenching race. Water rehydrates your body and bananas supply the mineral potassium that was depleted from the body during a race. Recent research has found that even those individuals who engage in moderate types of exercises need to be rehydrated with water and potassium after their exercise. Potassium is the mineral that works with the mineral called sodium to balance the fluids and electrolytes in your body. The main function of potassium is to maintain the electrolyte and fluid balance in your body. Potassium regulates your heartbeat and prevents muscle cramping and muscle fatigue and it may even protect you from hypertension and heart disease.

In a recent study conducted by the National Heart, Lung and Blood Institute, it was found that people with hypertension who consumed between 4,000 and 5,000 mg of potassium per day were able to lower their blood pressures in two to three weeks' time. This amount of potassium was easily obtained in the diet by consuming fruits, vegetables, whole grains, fish, nuts, beans, poultry and low-fat dairy products. These findings showed that potassium lowered blood pressure by regulating the heartbeat and by acting as a diuretic to get rid of excess fluid in the body. When excess fluid is released from the body, it causes a decrease in the fluid pressure, which is forced through the cardiovascular system, thus lowering the blood pressure. While potassium deficiency is seen mainly in strenuous prolonged exercise like running, potassium deficiency can also occur in moderate exercises, especially if you exercise in hot humid weather where excessive perspiration occurs. Always make sure to have a piece of fruit (banana, orange, etc.) with lots of water after you exercise.

The following foods are excellent sources of potassium:
1. Baked potato 800 mg.
2. Banana 500 mg.
3. Milk (8 ounces) 450 mg.
4. Yogurt (8 ounces) 400 mg.
5. Nectarines and oranges 300 mg.
6. Carrot (one medium) 300 mg.
7. Apricots, avocado, cantaloupe, honeydew, kiwi, beans, prunes, raisins, spinach and tomatoes all have between 225 and 275 mg of potassium.
8. Vegetable soup one cup can contain up to 1,500 mg of potassium depending on the amount of vegetables used.

FIT-STEP MYSTERY WALKING CLUES

1. Be alert. Be aware of your surroundings. Avoid an area that is unpopulated: deserted parks, trails, streets, parking lots, open fields.

2. Vary your route and time of day that you walk. Stick to daylight hours. Walk in familiar or well-populated areas. Plan your route beforehand.

3. If you feel uncomfortable in any area, turn back; follow your intuition. Let someone know where and when you walk. Carry a cell phone or change for a pay phone.

4. If possible, walk with a dog, a friend, or carry a stick, a walking cane, an umbrella, or just a branch for protection. Ignore strangers who ask you questions or call after you. Many stores now also carry walking sticks for dress or protection when you walk. These sticks can also help you climb hills if you are hiking and can act as a handy weapon if you have need to use one.

5. Be careful when you wear radio, CD or iPod earphones when walking since they may prevent you from hearing traffic or people coming up behind you. You can also place the earphones on the bony part of the skull (mastoid bone) directly behind each ear and you'll hear almost as well as if the earphones covered your ears. Otherwise keep the volume low to be aware of your surroundings.

6. Stay away from areas where people may hide: bushes, parked cars or trucks, alleyways, parking lots, etc. If you are threatened or are suspicious of anyone, run into a shopping center, apartment house, crowded street or just knock on someone's door.

7. Wear a whistle on a chain or carry a pocket noise alarm. Don't hesitate to use them even if you just suspect trouble. Wear light-colored clothing, especially if walking at dawn or dusk so that you are easily seen by traffic. When clothing is wet it appears darker than when it's dry, so be careful in rainy weather.

8. Never trust a moving vehicle! They'll never give you the right-of-way. Don't argue with a car. You'll be the loser.

9. Avoid overgrown or wooded areas and dark streets. Stay away from parked vehicles containing strangers.

10. If you become tired, stop and rest in a populated area (example: restaurant or a store).

11. If you're lost, call a friend or the police. Never hitchhike.

12. Be bright at night. Wearing reflective material on clothing and shoes while walking after dark or at dusk can mean the difference between a safe walk or a trip to the hospital. Reflective material will increase visibility as much as 200 to 750 feet. According to the American Committee of Accident and Poison Prevention, this reflective material could reduce night-time pedestrian deaths by 30-40%. Be bright at night; don't risk your inner light.

Walking For Fitness and Fun

1. Even though walking is the safest and most hazard-free exercise known to men and women, it is still essential that you have a complete physical examination by your family physician before starting your walking program.

2. Never exercise if you are injured or ill. Your body needs time to heal and recuperate from whatever ails you. Remember, you can't exercise through an injury or an illness. Many so-called fitness-nuts have tried this with disastrous results. For example, a strained muscle has been aggravated into a fractured bone or a simple cold has turned into pneumonia. Listen to your body.

3. Keep a record of your walking program. For example, how long did you walk today, and approximately how far did you go? Record the time and location and your impressions of the area in which you walked. Maybe it's an area you'd like to stay away from or one you'd like to explore again.

4. Record your weight only once every week to see if you are losing the amount of weight you'd like to lose, or if you are just walking to maintain your present weight. Remember walkers who want to maintain their present weight usually can have a bonus snack every day without gaining an ounce.

5. Don't expect results too soon. Whether it's fitness or weight-control that you're looking for, remember, "Rome wasn't built in a day and neither were you." Give your body time to adapt to your regular walking program.

6. Vary your walking program. Vary your walking times (morning, afternoon or evening) depending on your schedule.

7. Make your walking program convenient and flexible. The more adaptable you are to when and where you walk, the more likely you are to do it on a regular basis.

8. Either walk alone or with a friend or relative. Walking can be a social activity as well as an exercise. Spending time with someone you like or love can certainly add to the enjoyment of your walking program. Walking is one of the only exercises that lets you talk as you walk. If you are unable to talk because of shortness of breath then you're probably walking too fast.

9. Change your walking route every week or two. If near home or work, walk in a different direction, and observe, feel and smell new sights, sounds and odors on your new route. The road less traveled may be the most fun.

10. Take a walk-break instead of a coffee-break. Walking actually clears the mind and puts vitality and energy back into your body's walking machine. Coffee and a donut add caffeine and sugar to your body's sitting machine. Both the caffeine and sugar cause your insulin production to be increased, and following an initial rise in blood sugar, there is a sharp drop in your blood sugar from this excess insulin. So instead of coming back to work invigorated as you do from a walk break, you come back fatigued, light-headed and dizzy from a coffee and donut-break.

11. Wear a pedometer that keeps track of the miles that you walk. Some good computerized pedometers measure steps taken, distance traveled, calories burned, pace, heart rate and timed events.

12. Don't be afraid to take a break for a few days or even a week. Any exercise program, even one as easy and fun-filled as walking, can eventually become a little tiring. A few days' break from your schedule will give you a short breather so that you can return to your walking program with renewed interest and enthusiasm. Remember, you won't gain all of your weight back or get out of shape if you take an occasional break from your walking program.

MYSTERY CLUES FOR SHOES

1. Make sure the shoe fits properly. Shoes should be at least ½ to ¾ of an inch longer than your longest toe.

2. The toe section should be wide and high enough so as not to cause compression of your toes.

3. The shank (section between heel and ball of foot) should be wide enough with enough cushioning material to feel comfortable and springy.

4. The upper part of the shoe should be made of materials (soft leather, fabrics, suede, etc.) that are porous and flexible.

5. The sole and heel should be made of a thick, resilient material, which absorbs the shock of walking on a hard surface. And above all, make sure the shoes are comfortable.

6. Don't choose shoes by their size. Choose them by how they fit on your feet. (Remember, sizes vary among different shoe brands and styles.)

7. The size of your feet changes as you grow older. It's a good idea to have your feet re-measured regularly.

8. In most people, one foot is larger than the other. When you go shoe shopping, have both feet measured. Then select shoes that fit the largest foot.

9. Try to find shoes that conform as closely as possible to the shape of your foot.

10. If possible, try on shoes at the end of the day; that's when your feet are their largest and widest.

11. Stand up when you are trying on shoes. Make sure there is enough space between the end of the shoe and your longest toe. "Enough space" usually means that you should have room to put your finger between the end of your longest toe and the end of the shoe.

12. Make sure the ball of your foot fits comfortably into the widest part of the shoe.

13. Don't buy shoes that feel tight, hoping they will "stretch."

14. Select shoes that fit your heel comfortably and that allow a minimum amount of slippage.

15. Walk in the shoes that you want to buy to make sure that they fit and feel right.

Take a Happy Walk

Americans are walking again like never before. According to the President's Council on Physical Fitness report, walking is the single most popular adult exercise in America. With over 52 million adherents, the numbers are steadily increasing as men and women of all ages are walking for health, fitness and fun. Walking is an exercise whose time has finally come. Why not? It's easy, safe, fun and it makes you feel and look great.

Walking is something that two people, no matter how different their physical conditions, can do together. It is a companionable exercise in which you enjoy each other's company and at the same time get all the benefits of exercising. Walking is a great escape. You can get away from the phone, from the office, or from home for a little while, and take that needed time to relax. You can walk to think out a problem or walk to forget one. Walking acts as a tranquilizer to help us relax and it can work as a stimulant to give us energy. The late famous cardiologist Dr. Paul Dudley White said, "*A vigorous 3 mile walk will do more good for an unhappy but otherwise healthy adult than all the medicine and psychology in the world.*" Don't make the common mistake of thinking that walking is too easy to be a good exercise. On the contrary, walking is not only the safest, but it's the best exercise in the world. If you're overweight, then walking is your best choice since you won't be putting excessive stress on the ligaments, muscles, and joints.

I'm Giving Up! Exercise Is Boring

How many times have you heard someone or even perhaps yourself say, **"I'm giving up, exercise is boring!"** Over 65% of women and men who start an exercise program abandon it after 4-6 weeks. Surprising, isn't it? Not really! Initial enthusiasm is often quickly replaced by boredom. Most of the exercise equipment and athletic clothes quickly find their way into the recesses of the closet.

Walking, fortunately, is one of the only exercises that the majority of people stay with. The percentage of men and women who give up walking as a regular form of exercise is less than 25% of those who start on a walking program. Perhaps it's because walking doesn't require special equipment or clothing. Or perhaps it's because there are no clubs to join or dues to pay. Or perhaps it's just that most walkers are usually rugged individualists and are more determined than most to keep in good shape.

I think the real reason that walkers stay with their walking program is simply that walking is fun! And isn't that what an exercise should be? True, we all want physical fitness, good health, weight control and longevity. But we also want an escape from the stress of everyday living, and that's simply having fun. Walking provides a stress-free, fun-filled activity that we can do anyplace, anywhere, anytime whatsoever.

Stay Motivated

Most people who are overweight or not physically fit, are usually too embarrassed to join a gym. Joining a gym should be the last thing on your mind. All you have to do is take a brisk walk for 35 minutes six days per week, and you're on your way to losing weight and becoming physically fit. If you can't fit 35 minutes at one time into your daily schedule, then try to divide it into 2 or 3 sessions a day. Your weight-loss and fitness benefits will be exactly the same as one 35 minute daily walk.

Staying motivated is the key to any successful weight-loss and fitness program. Walking with a companion is one way to stay motivated. Also, by varying the route and location of your walk every couple of days will enjoy a fresh perspective on your daily walking exercise. You'll be exposed to new sights, sounds and smells, such as a park with pretty, fragrant flowers and beautiful trees. Also, you'll see different sections of the city or suburbs that you live or work in with a variety of new faces and places. It's easy to stay motivated with the Fit-Step Plan, since you will find new and exciting places to walk every day no matter what city or town that you live in.

Another sure-fire way to stay motivated when you walk is to vary the speed or intensity of walking during your walking exercise workout. For instance, speed up your walking pace for 30-60 seconds every 5 to 10 minutes during your 35 minute walk. You'll feel the extra energy pour into your body as you take in additional oxygen with your increased speed of walking. You'll also burn more calories as you speed up your walk, thus increasing your rate of weight-loss and physical fitness. Also, if you walk an extra 5 or 10 minutes a day, you will vary your daily exercise routine as you burn more calories for additional weight-loss and fitness.

You'll be able to stay motivated when you add the Strength-Training Exercises (Chapter 10), where you'll be walking for 35 minutes with light-weight, hand-held weight 2-3 times per week. These strength-training exercises help to build upper body muscles as you burn extra calories. By using different upper body muscles while walking with light-weight, hand-held weights, you'll feel the boost of energy surge throughout your body as your metabolic rate increases with this additional muscle activity. In fact, you'll have a double burst of calorie burning with the Fit-Step walking with weights plan. First you'll burn calories by the aerobic activity of walking and secondly you'll burn additional calories by building muscle tissue which actively burns calories. This double blast of calorie burning promotes maximum weight-loss, physical fitness and body shaping. This diet and fitness combo will get rid of those unwanted pounds for good.

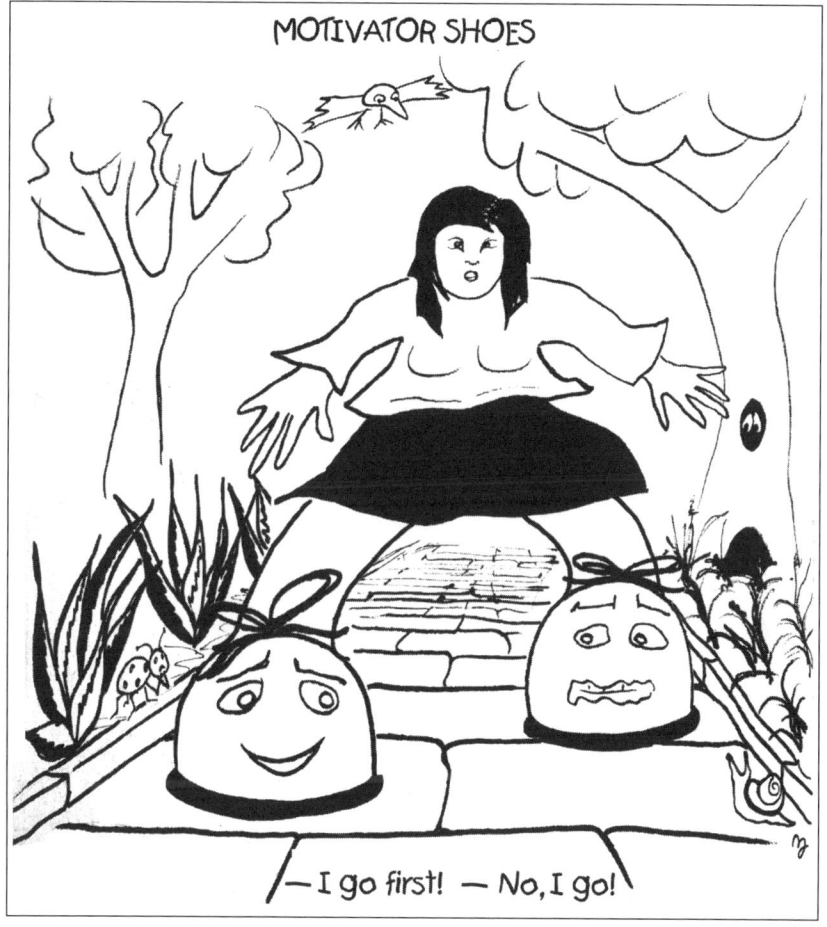

The Case of the Unwanted Pounds

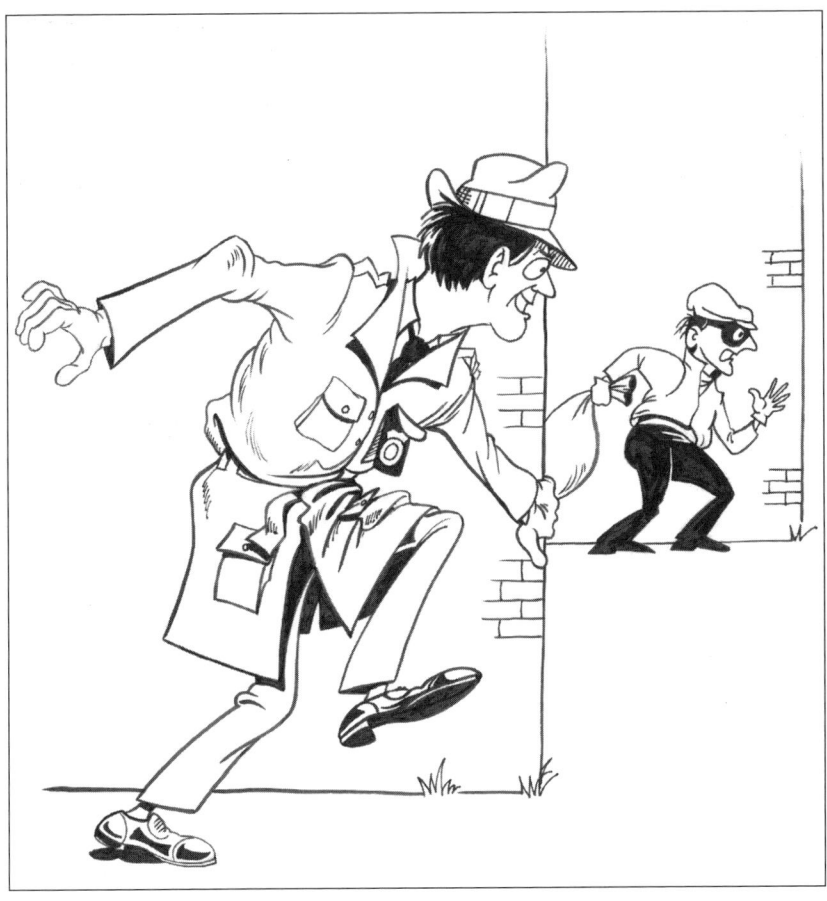

7

Detective Walker Stays Slim

Detective Adam Walker stealthfully followed his suspect, Lamont McIntyre, a known criminal, over the wet cobblestone winding streets of London, adjacent to the bay area. The air was wet and dank as they moved along in the fog, barely able to see but 10 feet in front of them. Walker was careful to keep as reasonable a distance as he could between them; however, because of the poor visibility it became necessary to follow his suspect at a closer, more dangerous range. It appeared that they were walking for considerably more than an hour, because before Walker realized, he was crossing the Piccadilly Circus area of town. Detective Walker, who was in relatively good shape from his daily walking program and healthy diet, was hardly winded at all. As they turned one corner after another, McIntyre looked back furtively as if he knew he was being followed. At one point he stopped and lit a cigarette and in the match's glow, looked around him more carefully to see if anyone was nearby. Once apparently satisfied, he proceeded along Fleet Street and then suddenly turned a corner and entered an alleyway behind a tobacco shop. He hesitated going any further, since the excess exertion of walking thus far had left him feeling fatigued and short of breath.

At this very moment, he regretted that he had neglected his health by not exercising regularly and eating a diet consisting of nothing but fried fish and chips and pints of ale. "Oh well," he thought, "It's too late to worry about that now." Lamont suddenly felt a tightness in his chest as he began to perspire profusely, and felt short of breath. He slowly proceeded into the alleyway and rested with his back up against the alley wall, which was not far from the street's entrance. McIntyre paused as his rapid breathing slowed and the discomfort in his chest abated. He drew his pistol from his topcoat and waited patiently for his pursuer, who he knew had to be Detective Walker. The detective had been following him doggedly for the past week, and Lamont knew there was no clear chance of escape. He would stand his ground and hope for the best by surprising his pursuer. A shadow approached the alleyway and he aimed his pistol at the very corner where the shadow appeared. It however was a woman who walked by the entrance to the alleyway, and McIntyre sighed and lowered his pistol.

As time passed, he actually believed he had finally eluded his pursuer, and then he began to slowly relax, when all of a sudden from the opposite end of the alley there loomed a formidable shadow with his pistol drawn, who said in a loud and clear voice, "Drop your weapon, McIntyre. It's Detective Walker, and you're under arrest." McIntyre had no intention of surrendering and vowed never to spend another day in jail. He quickly raised and aimed his pistol toward the detective and was about to fire, when he suddenly saw a flash of light and felt and heard a shattering sound in his right shoulder, which caused him to drop his pistol and cry out in severe pain. "Stay where you are," shouted Walker, "or the next bullet will be in your chest."

McIntyre slid slowly down with his back up against the alley wall, and finally sitting on the alley floor with his legs splayed out said, "Walker, you'll never take me alive," as he slowly reached down with his other hand, located the pistol, and aimed and fired quickly at the detective. His shot went wide of its mark, and then he suddenly felt and heard a thunderous explosion in his chest. He lay still against the wall, as he watched his life's blood flow gradually away from his body into the dank sewer drain nearby, and then he was still forevermore. As the detective slowly approached the body he said softly, "Lamont, you should have stayed in better shape, if you wanted to live longer, not to mention the fact that you should never have resorted to a life of crime."

Detective Adam Walker of Scotland Yard was known to have exercised regularly with a daily walking program, worked out with light weights several days per week and had healthy eating habits. He was slightly over six feet tall and his body build was both lithe and muscular. He was in considerably better shape than most of his constituents, and was able to keep his weight within a normal range because of his regular daily walking routine. Whenever he noticed that he gained a few pounds, he would just rev-up his exercise program by walking for another 30 to 60 minutes daily. He found this to be an extremely effective method for quick weight loss. He often found that when he had to follow a suspect, he was often required to walk for long distances at a time, as we have seen demonstrated in the above case. He noted that on these occasions he was able to maintain his normal body weight quite easily.

Just like Detective Walker's method for quick weight-loss, it's important for us to realize that faster weight loss can only result from walking for longer periods of time than just 35 minutes daily. In this chapter we will deal with quick weight-loss walking plans that allow you to lose weight at a faster rate, than the weight that you would ordinarily lose on your regular walking program. These quick weight-loss plans involve walking briskly for longer distances and for longer periods of time, than you would ordinarily walk on the standard Diet Fit-Step Plan. As Detective Walker stated, "You should stay in good shape by walking briskly on a regular basis, eat a healthy diet, and most assuredly avoid a life of crime."

The Fat Formula

The latest report from the National Institute of Health again confirmed that obesity is a major health risk. The evidence is strong that obesity not only shortens life, but actually affects the quality of life also. Almost 20 percent of Americans are overweight. How can you tell if you're one of them? It's simple—just follow the **fat formula** for your normal weight:

Females – 100 lbs. for the first 5 feet in height, plus 5 lbs. for each additional inch. Example: 5'2" = 110 lbs.

Males – 106 lbs. for the first 5 feet in height, plus 6 lbs. for each additional inch. Example: 5' 9" = 160 lbs.

BMI

Body mass index (BMI) is a new measurement of your weight, related to your height. It is another way to assess body fat in relation to your height. The BMI is a complicated mathematical formula based on your weight in pounds and your height in inches. It's much easier to consult BMI tables on the Internet or in health magazines than it is to try to figure out this mathematical formula yourself. Generally the BMI also rates your risk of heart disease depending on your body mass index. The following is a general chart **(Table I),** which indicates if you're overweight and your potential risk of heart disease.

TABLE I

BMI	WEIGHT	HEART DISEASE RISK
18.5-24.9	Normal	None
25.0-29.9	Overweight	Increased
30.0-34.0	Obese	High
35.0-39.9	Obese	Very High
40.0 or greater	Extremely Obese	Extremely High

If you flunk the fat formula or the BMI, then you really need to start walking-off weight using the **Quick Weight-Loss Walking Plans.** The increased medical risks for being overweight are: hypertension, heart attacks, strokes, diabetes, arthritis, cancer of all types, and increased surgical risks if you happen to need an operation. These risks seem to be even worse if most of your weight is carried in the upper body (chest, hips and particularly the abdomen) rather than in the buttocks and legs.

DIETS DON'T REALLY WORK

Consumer Reports polled 95,000 subscribers who tried to lose weight over the last three to five years. Over 19,000 subscribers used commercially supervised diet programs, and the rest tried to lose weight on their own. The results of both groups were similar, in that dieters lost an average of 10-12 pounds while on their respective diets. The discouraging news, however, is that most of the respondents to this survey regained almost one-half of their weight loss in the first three to six months after ending the diet program, and two-thirds of the weight was regained in two years. Only 20% of these dieters were able to keep off two-thirds of the weight they had lost for more than a two-year period. Many of these commercial diet programs cost an average of $65-70 per week—a pretty hefty price to pay for a temporary weight loss plan.

Diets by themselves don't work! It doesn't appear that we're getting any thinner despite all of the diet books, diet centers and health clubs. So what's the answer to this timeless question? Walking, of course! Walkers by and large are the least overweight segment of any population group. This fact has been verified in hundreds of medical studies.

You can then actually lose weight by just walking. When you walk at a brisk speed of 3.5 mph for one hour every day, you will burn up 350 calories each day. Therefore, if you walk one hour a day for 10 days, you will burn up to a total 3,500 calories. Since there are 3,500 calories in each pound of fat, by walking one hour daily for 10 days, you will lose one pound of fat. You will continue to lose one pound of body fat every time you complete 10 hours of walking at a speed of 3.5 mph. It works every time!

On the regular Fit-Step:35 minute plan, you will walk 35 minutes, six days per week and burn approximately 235 calories (3.5 mph) every 35 minutes. On the Quick Weight Loss Walking Plans, we will just be increasing the walking time to **45 or more minutes every day.** The longer you walk, the more calories you'll burn, and that's where the **Quick Weight-Loss Walking Plans** come in to play.

Want to Lose Weight Faster?

Most women are more likely to perceive themselves as fat, whereas in reality, men are more likely to be overweight. In a recent Harris poll of over 1,200 women and men nationwide, the findings were as follows:

- Over 50% of women considered themselves overweight, compared to 38% of men.
- 65% of the men were actually overweight, compared with 62% of the woman.
- Almost 40% of those people surveyed stated that they were on a diet.
- 60% of those surveyed were overweight, which was exactly the same percentage as last year's survey.
- More than 50% of those surveyed felt they weren't getting enough exercise.

"I Don't Really Eat That Much!"

The question I get asked most often from patients about being overweight is, "How come I keep gaining weight? I don't really eat that much." Well, the truth of the matter is that we get heavier as we get older because our physical activity tends to decrease even though our food intake stays the same. The only way to beat the battle of the bulge is to burn those unwanted pounds away. Walking actually **burns calories**. The following table will give you an idea as to the energy expended in walking, which is actually the number of calories per minute or per hour (**TABLE II**).

TABLE II

Walking Speed	Calories Burned/Minute	Calories Burned/30 Minutes	Calories Burned/Hour
Slow Speed (2 mph)	3-4	105-130	210-260
Moderate Speed (3 mph)	4-5	130-160	260-330
Brisk Speed (3.5 mph)	**5-6**	**160-180**	**320-380**
Fast Speed (4 mph)	6-7	180-220	380-440
Race Walking (5 mph)	7-8	220-260	440-520

A pound of body fat contains approximately 3,500 calories. When you eat 3,500 more calories than your body actually needs, it stores up that pound as body fat. If you reduce your intake by 3,500 calories, you will lose a pound. It doesn't make any difference how long it takes your body to store or burn these 3,500 calories. The result is always the same. You either gain or lose one pound of body fat, depending on how long it takes you to accumulate or burn up 3,500 calories.

QUICK WEIGHT-LOSS WALKING

The Regular Fit-Step: 35 Minute Plan was based on walking at a brisk pace (3.5 mph) for 35 minutes six days per week, combined with the **Diet-Step Plan**: **35/35 Plan.** This weight-loss program is based upon the number of calories burned by the combination of dieting and walking. Walking at 3.5 miles per hour is a speed that can be maintained for a long duration without causing stress, strain or fatigue. We are not recommending slow walking (1 to 2 miles/hr) since is not useful in burning calories. Nor are we suggesting fast walking (4-5 miles/hr.), which is too fast to be continued for long periods of time without tiring you. And we certainly are not recommending race walking (5 to 6 miles/hr), which is worthless as a permanent weight reduction plan, and has all of the same hazards and dangers that running has. **On the Quick Weight-Loss Walking Plans noted below, you will be walking for 45 or more minutes every day of the week.**

By following **The Quick Weight-Loss Walking Plans,** you will lose additional weight by actually walking off more weight. This faster weight loss occurs because you will be walking for 45 minutes or more every day. The following Quick Weight-Loss Plans have been designed for faster weight-loss than the weight that you lose on the Diet-Step & Fit-Step Plan.

By following any one of these four Quick Weight-Loss Walking Plans, you will be able to lose more weight than you can lose on the Diet-Step/Fit-Step combination plan alone. **This additional weight-loss occurs because you will be walking for longer periods of time (45 or more minutes every day).** Remember, it's easy to lose more weight and look your best by just walking more every day. You can then actually lose weight by just walking. When you walk at a speed of 3.5 mph for one hour every day, you will burn up **350 calories each day.**

1. QUICK WEIGHT-LOSS WALKING PLAN #1

Walk 45 minutes every day and you'll lose one additional pound every 15 days.

If you walk for 45 minutes every day you will burn up 3,500 calories in 15 days. Since there are 3,500 calories in each pound of fat, every time you burn up 3,500 calories by walking, you will lose a pound of body fat.

2. QUICK WEIGHT-LOSS WALKING PLAN #2

Walk one hour every day and lose one additional pound every 10 days.

Since it takes 10 hours of walking at 3.5 mph to burn up 3,500 calories or one pound, if you walk for **one hour every day,** you will **lose one additional pound every 10 days.** By following this plan you can actually **lose 3 extra pounds every month**.

3. QUICK WEIGHT-LOSS WALKING PLAN #3

Walk 1½ hours every day and lose one additional pound every 7 days.

For those of you who want to lose weight even faster, you can walk for **1½ hours every day or 45 minutes twice daily**. By walking a total of **1½ hours every day of the week** you will be able to speed up the walking-off-weight on this plan. When you walk 1½ hours every day, you will burn up 525 calories each day or 3,675 calories per week. You can see that you will lose a pound a week on this plan with a few extra (175 calories) to spare.

4. QUICK WEIGHT-LOSS WALKING SNACK PLAN #4

Snack on your favorite food—calorie free.

Let's say your weight is just where you'd like it to be, but you don't want to gain another ounce. Or say your weight is nowhere near what you would like it to be, but you really can't afford to gain another pound. How about a slice of cake, French fries, a cone of ice cream, a slice of pizza, a hamburger or a glass of wine?

With the **Quick Weight-Loss Walking Snack Plan** you have the perfect method that allows you to cheat without paying the price. Eat your favorite snack food, consult the following table **(TABLE III)** and walk the number of minutes listed in order to burn up the extra calories you've cheated on. The following table shows how many minutes of walking at a brisk pace (3½ mph) are necessary to burn up the caloric value of those foods listed.

If your favorite snack food is not listed on the following table, you can easily figure out the time you have to burn off your snack's calories. **Look up the number of calories of your favorite snack food and divide by the number 6.** This answer will give you the number of minutes it takes to walk off your snack. The number 6 comes from the fact that walking at a brisk pace (3.5 mph) burns approximately 6 calories per minute. Example: hamburger and roll = 438 calories. Divide 6 into 438 and you get the number 73. It will therefore take you 73 minutes to walk off this snack.

TABLE III

Quick Weight-Loss Walking Snack Plan
(Time Required to Walk Off Snacks)

Snacks	Time Required to Walk Off Snacks
American cheese (1 slice)	16 minutes
apple (medium)	15 minutes
apple juice (6 oz.)	17 minutes
bagel (1)	23 minutes
banana (medium)	16 minutes
beer (12 oz.)	30 minutes
bologna sandwich	50 minutes
candy bar (1 oz.)	45 minutes
cake (1 slice pound)	63 minutes
chocolate bar/nuts (1 oz.)	28 minutes
cheese crackers (6)	35 minutes
cheese steak (½)	55 minutes

chicken, fried (3 pieces)	50 minutes
chocolate cookies (3)	25 minutes
corn chips (small pack)	33 minutes
doughnut (jelly)	40 minutes
frankfurter & roll	50 minutes
French fries (3 oz.)	50 minutes
hamburger (4 oz.) and roll	73 minutes
ice cream cone	30 minutes
ice cream sandwich	35 minutes
ice cream sundae	75 minutes
milk shake, choc. (8 oz.)	42 minutes
muffin, blueberry	25 minutes
orange juice (6 oz.)	16 minutes
peanut butter crackers (6)	50 minutes
peanuts, in shell (2 oz.)	37 minutes
pie, apple (1 slice)	46 minutes
pizza (1 slice)	40 minutes
potato chips (small pack)	33 minutes
pretzels (hard – 3 small)	30 minutes
pretzels (soft – 1 Superpretzel®)	30 minutes
shrimp cocktail (6 small)	18 minutes
soda-cola (12 oz.)	24 minutes
tuna fish sandwich	41 minutes
wine, Chablis (4 oz.)	14 minutes
whiskey, rye (1 oz.)	17 minutes

EATING AND EXERCISE

As food enters your stomach, the heart pumps a significant quantity of blood into the stomach to aid in the digestive process. This does not pose a problem when you are at rest, but if you decide to exercise immediately after eating, then there is a conflict of interest. The stomach now has to compete with the exercising muscles for the blood it needs for digestion. If the exercise gets vigorous then digestion is arrested and you begin to feel bloated and develop abdominal cramps. Exercise should therefore begin after a meal has passed through the stomach and small intestines. This takes approximately 2 hours after ingesting a large meal and from 45-60 minutes after eating a smaller meal. However, as you'll note below, you can actually begin to walk approximately 30 to 45 minutes after a small meal which helps to aid digestion and weight-loss.

Foods high in saturated fat and unhealthy fatty protein are not efficient foods for energy production and tend to store excess fat in the body's fat cells. Foods that are high in refined sugar like cakes, candy and pies can trigger an excess insulin response if they are eaten immediately before exercise. This means that the excess insulin produced as a result of the high sugar content of food, combined with the exertion of exercise, could drop the blood sugar rapidly. This could result in weakness, muscle cramps and even fainting. On the other hand, foods that are higher in complex carbohydrates (whole-grain foods, vegetables, fruits) and healthy protein (lean meats, fish, white meat of chicken and turkey; non-fat dairy products; nuts and seeds) tend to be absorbed slowly, thus avoiding the insulin spikes and the drops of blood sugar. These foods are efficient energy producers and burn calories steadily, so that no excess fat is stored in the body's fat cells.

On the other hand, fasting for long periods prior to exercise is in itself counterproductive. In order to replenish the energy stores (glycogen) in the liver and muscles, it is necessary to eat several hours before exercising. When you fast, you deplete these energy stores, and exercise then becomes difficult and tiring without adequate fuel storage reserves for energy.

So what does this all have to do with walking and eating? Very little, if anything. Most of these rules of digestion apply to strenuous and vigorous exercise with relation to mealtime. They do, however, affect us somewhat with regards to our walking program. The most important fact to be learned from this discussion on digestive physiology is that it is essential that you don't walk immediately after eating, especially if you've consumed a relatively large meal (which you shouldn't be eating in the first place). This puts a strain on the cardiovascular system and can even deprive the heart of its own essential blood supply, particularly if you exercise vigorously immediately after eating (which you shouldn't be doing in the second place).

However, walking at a moderate pace of 3½ mph, approximately 30 to 45 minutes after a small meal can actually aid in digestion, by nudging the foodstuffs gently along the digestive tract. This in no way competes for the blood in the digestive tract, since your walking muscles do not require nearly as much as strenuously exercising muscles require. In fact, the gentle art of walking allows oxygen to be evenly distributed to all of the body's internal organs, which in this particular case is the digestive tract. You will burn more fat calories as you walk after eating. If however, you feel tired or short of breath, or develop any type of pain, stop and rest. If the pain or any other symptoms persists, then see your doctor immediately.

Recent studies indicate a three-fold advantage for dieters who walk before and after meals. As we have previously seen, walking before eating slows down our appetite-control center in the brain and makes us less hungry. Secondly, walking at any time burns calories directly as we walk. And thirdly, new studies in exercise physiology have shown that walking anywhere from 30-45 minutes after eating a small meal will actually burn 10-15% more calories than walking on an empty stomach. This is explained by a term called the **thermic dynamic action of food**. What this means is that the actual digestion of food products combined with the gentle action of walking results in a higher metabolic rate, thus burning more calories per hour. Also, because of this increase in your basal metabolic rate, your body actually continues to burn more calories after you walk, than it does at rest alone.

EXERCISE INCREASES YOUR APPETITE: RIGHT?—WRONG!

Another myth regarding diet and exercise is that exercise stimulates the appetite. So after you exercise you're hungry, and then you eat more, and you cancel out any calories you burned during exercise. Right? Wrong! Contrary to popular belief, walking actually decreases your appetite. It does this by several mechanisms which are described as follows:

1. **Walking burns fat** rather than carbohydrates and therefore does not drop the blood sugar precipitously. Strenuous exercises and calorie-reduction diets both drop the blood sugar rapidly, and it is this low blood sugar that stimulates your appetite and makes you hungry. Walking on the other hand is a more moderate type of exercise and consequently burns fats slowly rather than carbohydrates quickly. This results in the blood sugar remaining constant. And when the blood sugar remains level, you do not feel hungry.

2. Walking also **increases the resting basal metabolic rate (BMR)**. This basal metabolic rate refers to the calories your body burns at rest in order to produce energy. When you go on a calorie restriction diet, your BMR slows. This is because your body assumes that the reduction in calories is the result of starvation and your body wants to burn fewer calories so you won't starve to death. The body has no way of knowing that you're on a diet. This is also one of the reasons that you don't continue to lose weight on a calorie reduction diet. The body prevents this excess weight loss by lowering its BMR, so that you stop losing weight even though you are eating the same number of calories that you ate in the beginning of your diet.

3. Walking regulates the brain's appetite control center (**appestat**), which controls hunger pangs. Too little exercise causes your appetite to increase by stimulating the appestat to make you hungry. Walking slows the appestat down, decreasing your hunger pangs.

4. Walking **redirects the blood supply** away from your stomach, towards the exercising muscles. With less blood supplied to the stomach, your appetite is reduced.

5. When you combine the **Diet-Step Plan: 35 Gm Fat/ 35 Gm Fiber,** with 35 minutes of walking on the **Fit-Step: 35 Minute Walking Plan**, the walking component powers up your basal metabolic rate, and causes you to burn more calories than if you were just following the diet alone. So walking prevents the BMR from decreasing and burning fewer calories, as when you only diet. The result: less hunger and more calories burned when you walk every day.

Fast Eaters Gain Weight Faster

Researchers from Osaka University in Japan studied the eating habits and body mass of approximately 3500 men and women between the ages of 30 and 69. Those individuals who ate quickly or ate until they felt full doubled their risk of being overweight. Those people who had both of the above bad habits were more than three times as likely to be overweight. Being overweight means that you are at higher risk for developing hypertension, heart disease, strokes, and even certain forms of cancer. This study emphasizes that if you are interested in losing weight, you should eat meals at a slower pace and stop eating before you feel completely full.

Boost Metabolism to Burn Calories

Some people are born with a high rate of metabolism. They essentially burn almost all of the food that they eat, and actually have difficulty gaining weight, no matter how many calories they consume. They, however, are the exception to the rule. Most of us aren't so lucky, and we have to work in order to boost our metabolic rate.

Regular exercise is the most important component in the metabolism boosting equation. The basic weight maintenance equation is: *your weight is determined by how much you eat and how much you exercise.* When you exercise regularly like a daily walking program, you take care of the movement side of the equation. This is actually the key component to preventing weight gain. By exercising more frequently you will burn calories at a faster rate, and the calorie burning will continue even after you've stopped exercising. If the exercise component of the metabolic equation is greater than the amount of food that you eat, then you will lose weight because of your increased metabolic rate. When your exercise routine is convenient and enjoyable, you'll have greater success in your exercise program. Nothing could be easier and more convenient than a regular aerobic exercise walking program. You can do it anywhere, anyplace and any time. You can walk alone or with a friend, and best of all, you do not have to join a gym to get the benefits of an aerobic exercise walking program.

Overeating and snack foods will slow down your metabolism, and cause you to gain weight. Stress, emotional eating and boredom all play a role in overeating high carbohydrate and high fat foods. If you're really hungry for snack foods, choose healthy foods to avoid excess calories, which pile on the unwanted pounds. Overeating can be linked to one very important factor: **portion control**. Studies have shown that overweight people who controlled their portion sizes were more likely to take weight off and keep it off permanently. Weight gain is a gradual process, and sneaks up on you day by day. So it's important for you to eat sensibly and avoid unhealthy snacking and be extremely mindful of portion control.

Surprisingly, there are some foods that can actually help you to boost your metabolism and burn calories. Some of these metabolism boosting foods include whole grains (breads, cereals, and pastas), legumes, beans, nuts, seeds, fresh fruits, and omega-3 fatty foods like salmon and flax seed. These foods provide a steady and constant source of fuel for your body. Your body's metabolism will then increase its calorie burning process throughout the day, and provide you with enough energy to carry on your daily functions.

Strenuous exercise after a large meal causes the increased blood supply in the stomach and intestinal tract to be diverted to the exercising muscles. This puts a strain on the cardiovascular system, especially in anyone who has a heart or circulatory problem. A calm walk, on the other hand, approximately 35-40 minutes after eating a small meal, does not stress the cardiovascular system and burns many of the excess calories that you should not have eaten in the first place. It's far better to get up and walk away from that big meal before you overstuff your face. When you physically walk away from the table you are removing yourself from temptation, but even more importantly, you are allowing the fullness control center in your brain to catch up to what's really going on in your stomach. You are actually full, but you don't know it yet. Remember, eating less and walking more are the only two ways to lose weight effectively, or, to put it another way—walk more and eat less!

Many studies have clearly documented the weight-loss effects of exercise. Even more important is that the weight loss caused by walking is almost all due to the burning of body fat, not carbohydrates. This weight loss or weight maintenance can be continued indefinitely as long as you walk regularly. You are literally walking off weight. Not only does walking before meals decrease your appetite, but recent studies show that walking approximately 30-45 minutes after eating increases the metabolic body rate to burn away calories at a faster rate. It appears, then, that walking after eating is another way to lose additional pounds. Never walk, however, immediately after a large meal is ingested.

This burning of calories at a faster rate has been explained as a combination of the energy expended from walking and the calories burned from the ingestion of food itself. This is called the **Thermic Effect of Food** or the **Specific Dynamic Action**. We burn more calories as we eat because the energy metabolism of the body increases 5-10%. This doesn't mean that the more you eat the more calories you'll burn. But it is a good reason for walking 35-40 minutes after small meals for additional weight loss. If you want to lose weight faster, walk for 35 minutes before meals to reduce your appetite and walk an additional 35 minutes after small meals to burn more calories.

WALKING BURNS BODY FAT NOT CARBOHYDRATES

If you just count calories or worse yet carbohydrates, your chances of losing weight are almost zero. Walking is the only certain way towards permanent weight reduction. The majority of obese people are much less active than most thin people. It is their sedentary lifestyle that accounts for their excess weight and not their overeating.

If you want to lose weight permanently, then the energy burned during your exercise should come from fats and not from carbohydrates. **During the first 35-40 minutes of moderate exercise (walking), only ⅓ of the energy burned comes from carbohydrates while ⅔ comes from body fats.** During short bursts of strenuous exercise, ⅔ of the energy burned comes from carbohydrates and only ⅓ from body fat. It stands to reason, then, that a continuous exercise like walking, which burns primarily body fats, is a lot better for permanent weight reduction than short spurts of strenuous exercise (examples: jogging, calisthenics, racquetball, etc.).

If you increase the duration of your walking from your regular daily 35 minutes to 45-60 minutes, you will burn more energy from body fats, resulting in faster weight-loss. Once you've lost your weight, you will maintain your weight better by walking 35 minutes every day than by doing calisthenics or running for 15-20 minutes. This occurs because you will be burning a higher proportion of body fats rather than carbohydrates.

THE MYSTERY OF 10,000 STEPS

In a recent study, researchers have discovered that walking approximately 10,000 steps a day is a threshold for physical fitness and weight loss. The women studied in this group wore pedometers every day to measure the number of steps that they took daily. After a six week period, the women who averaged 10,000 steps or more daily were found to have 35% less body fat and had lost 3-4 inches in their waist and hip measurements, compared to those women who took less than 6,000 steps per day. There are several other similar studies that have shown that both men and women who walked 10,000 steps or more daily, not only lost weight but also had significantly lower blood pressures.

Six thousand steps means that you've walked approximately 3 miles. This appears to be the average number of steps that most active adults walk in a day, provided that they're not desk-bound for 8 hours. In order to add another 4,000 steps per day to this 6,000 step average, it would be necessary to walk for an additional 30 minutes a day. So here again we have more concrete proof, that walking 35 minutes a day in addition to your regular activity is a great way to lose weight, get firm and fit and boost energy. All that you need to do is start and continue a regular 35 minute walking program six days per week and you will reach your target weight in no time at all.

Buy an inexpensive pedometer. It doesn't have to be a computer-driven model which really does nothing more than a regular pedometer. All it has to do is count your steps while you're walking. Pedometers come with an adjustable feature so that you can set your stride length into the pedometer's memory. It's easy enough to measure the length of your stride while walking by using a tape measure when you start out. Some pedometers do it automatically; others require that you set the stride length. A really good computerized pedometer will measure the steps you've taken, the distance walked, the calories burned and your heart rate. However, an inexpensive pedometer works just as well. It's a great way to measure the number of steps that you've taken and the distance that you've walked.

If you're just starting your Diet Fit-Step Plan, wear the pedometer for a few days to get the average steps per day. Then add approximately 500 additional steps each day until you hit the mystery number of 10,000 steps. This is the number of steps that is supposed to be required for cardiovascular fitness. However, 10,000 steps is really a myth. It's the time that you walk each day and the consistency of your walking program that really is the key to weight loss, body-shaping and cardiovascular fitness. You may find that you're taking 15,000 steps or 750 steps per day to achieve fitness. The pedometer is more of a gimmick to give people something to hang their hats on while walking. If you like to use it, by all means do so, otherwise it's really not necessary on the Diet Fit-Step Plan. You'll be getting all of the fitness and weight loss benefits you need by walking briskly for 35 minutes, 6 days a week at approximately 3½ miles per hour, whether you use a pedometer or not.

In reality, it doesn't matter if you walk exactly 10,000 steps a day. All that really matters on the Diet Fit-Step Plan, is that you walk for 35 minutes six days per week, and walk with light-weight, hand-held weights three days per week, for maximum weight-loss and fitness. With this plan, combined with all of your daily activities, you will certainly walk many more steps daily, than the so-called mystery number of 10,000 steps.

The Detective's Walking Tips

A. Stay well-hydrated.

Our bodies are composed of approximately 60% water. Water regulates almost every body metabolic process. Water regulates the digestion and absorption of foods and the elimination of toxins in the bloodstream. It also helps the blood flow to supply oxygen, energy and nutrients to every cell, tissue and organ in your body, including all of your muscles and your brain. Water also aids your metabolism in keeping your body temperature normal. If you are overheated, the body produces sweat to let you know that you need to replace the water that is lost from your body. This is especially true if you're a detective who's following someone for a long distance.

You can lose almost a quart of water while exercising. You should have at least a glass of water 20-30 minutes before exercise and another glass of water when you are finished with your exercise. It's a good idea to have a bottle of water with you while you're walking and you should take sips regularly while walking. Don't wait until you are thirsty. One of the very first signs of dehydration is fatigue. You can purchase water bottle safety clips that can be attached to your clothing or belt while walking. Also, on the 3 days per week that you are walking with weights, you can occasionally switch the one pound hand-held weights for two 12 ounce bottles of water in each hand. You can drink alternately from each bottle as you walk. Use the water bottles like the hand-held weights for upper body strength training exercises.

Stay away from so-called power drinks, sodas, fruit punch, lemonade and any drinks with added sugar. Many of these so-called power drinks contain caffeine, which can actually cause dehydration in addition to raising your blood pressure and heart rate.

A 2009 study of 810 adults published by the *American Journal of Clinical Nutrition* reported that cutting back on liquid calories may be the quickest route to shed unwanted pounds. Participants lost more weight cutting down on liquid calories than they did cutting down on solid calories over a period of 18 months. The theory proposed why liquid calories are weightier than solid calories, is that people do not chew beverages, which results in a lower hormone response that signal fullness. In other words, people still are hungry after drinking sweetened beverages. Also, the sweeteners that are added to these beverages may also promote fat storage and increase your appetite.

B. Clothing and shoes.

In warm weather, wear breathable material that keeps your body cool. In cooler weather, layer-up your clothing to stay warm and comfortable. Socks should be padded, cotton to absorb moisture. If your feet get too sweaty or you are prone to form foot blisters, then look into acrylic socks.

Remember that socks can affect your shoe size, so wear the type of socks you'll be wearing while walking when you try on new walking shoes. Make sure you have a comfortable walking shoe with enough wiggle room for your toes. You also want good cushioning throughout the length of the shoe. Be careful about a shoe with too high an arch support, which can throw off your stride and can cause your feet to ache. Try the shoe on in the store, and walk around a while to make sure that the shoe feels comfortable.

Air cell insoles can add comfort to your feet while walking. By adding thin, extra cushioning to your walking shoes, you will walk with more spring and energy in your step. These insoles add high performance to any walking shoe.

Detectives should always wear shoes with a lot of insole cushioning and a sturdy outer sole, in order to absorb the impact from walking on hard surfaces. This will also insure that their footsteps are quiet, in order to prevent suspects from knowing that they're being followed. Also they should wear properly fitted shoes with good support and cushioning in order to keep their feet comfortable and free of foot injuries. In earlier times, policemen were called "flat-foots," because they didn't have the advantage of walking with any of the newer, more modern types of padded, support shoes.

C. Increase Fitness by Walking Up Hills

To burn calories at a faster rate, try walking up an incline, such as a moderate grade hill for a short period of time, say five or ten minutes. Walking up the hill will increase your metabolic rate and you will burn calories at a faster rate than by just walking on a flat surface. You will notice a faster heart rate and faster breathing as you walk up the incline.

However, you must be in relatively good shape to walk up hills. This means that you should have been on your 35 minute daily walking program for at least six to eight weeks before you attempt to walk up hills. If you become tired or short of breath then stop and rest. You should be able to walk up slightly graded inclines without any discomfort if you are in reasonably good shape. If, however, you find that walking up hills seem too difficult or tires you too easily, then continue your regular walking program on flat surfaces.

Steep hills should definitely be avoided because the risks of ligament and tendon injuries are much more frequent when walking up steep inclines. In particular, it is the down hill descent that makes you more prone to ankle and knee injuries because on the descent your stride is uneven and you start to descend faster because of gravity, so that you have to actually drag your heels into the dirt in order to prevent you from accelerating too fast. If your goal is to burn calories at a faster rate and you feel relatively comfortable walking up mild to moderately graded hills, you can make hill climbing a part of your weekly walking program, say for five or ten minutes on two or three days per week.

Remember too that walking up uneven, slightly graded hills can cause leg muscle fatigue and muscle cramps, so be sure to stop walking if your legs cramp up and switch to walking on a flat surface. Hills are only necessary if you feel that you have to speed up your metabolism to burn more calories. Otherwise, you can get the same fat burning boost by just walking on flat surfaces for a longer period of time without the hazards and/or dangers of climbing hills.

D. Efficient walking

Efficient walking will help to prevent injuries and burn more calories in less time. Follow the standard detective's walking tips:

1. Relax your upper arms and shoulders as you walk.
2. Walk while standing straight. Don't lean backwards or forwards.
3. Take small to medium quick strides, rather than long, slow motion ones.
4. Hit the ground first with your heel, and then roll your foot forward, and then push off with your toes.
5. Bend your arms at an approximate 90° angle, and keep them close to the side of your body. Close your hands in loose, not tight, fists.
6. Swing your arms forward and backwards in rhythm with your walking stride. Keep both elbows close to your body while using your arm motion.
7. Walk with your chin level to the ground. Don't look up or down. Focus on the horizon or whatever else is directly ahead of you, like a criminal suspect.
8. Detectives rarely if ever wear pedometers, since they can produce noise and may also get in the way when pursuing a suspect.

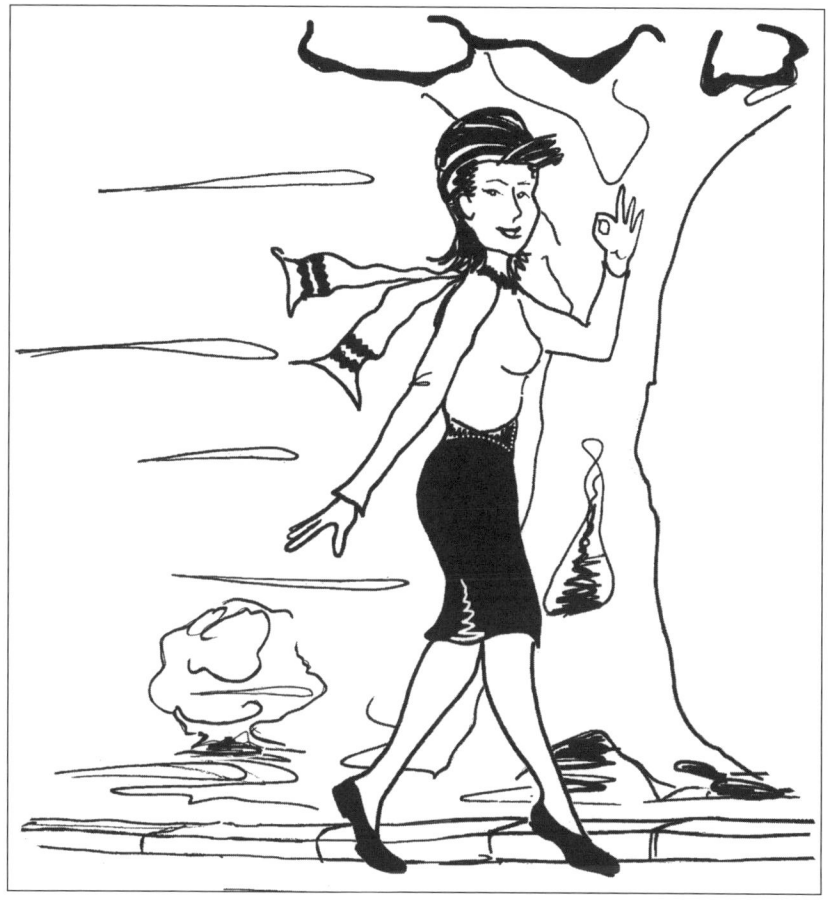

"It's no mystery. Walking keeps me slim."

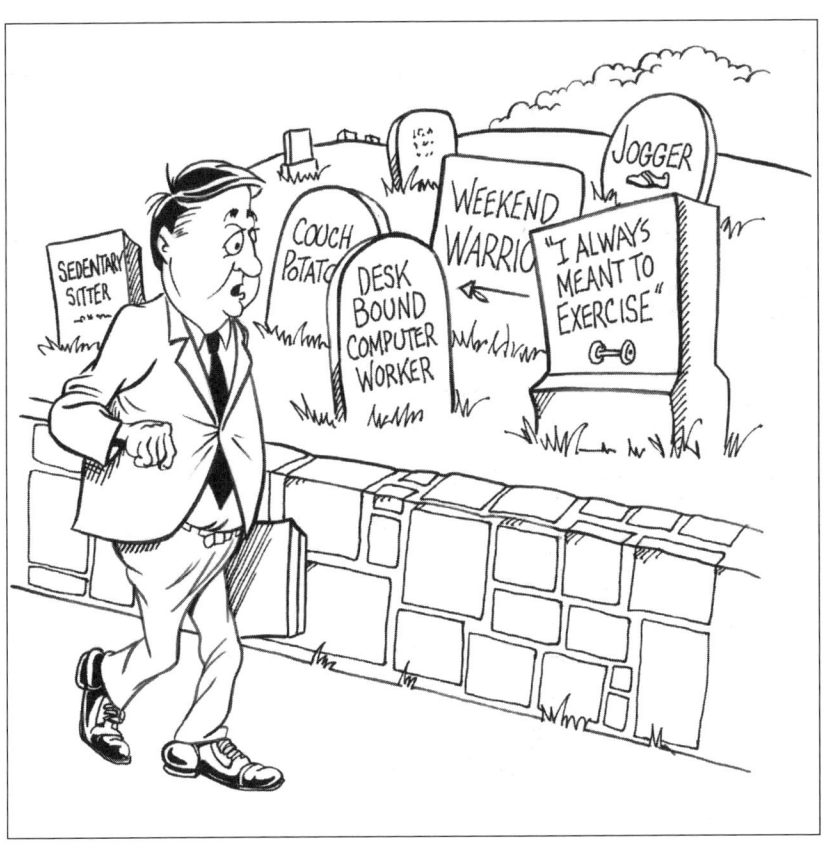

8

Walk, Don't Die!

It is a well known fact that a regular exercise program, like an aerobic walking program is beneficial in weight loss, fitness and good health. Walkers by in large live longer than any segment of the population in this country and in countries throughout the world. Walking helps to prevent obesity, heart attacks, strokes, hypertension, diabetes, some forms of cancer, arthritis, osteoporosis, degenerative diseases of aging including Alzheimer's disease, among many other diseases and disorders. The life expectancy for people who do not exercise has been shown to be at least 10 to 15 years less than for people who exercise regularly. A regular aerobic walking program is the perfect exercise to supply your body with a continuous stream of life-giving and life-sustaining oxygen.

Oxygen from the atmosphere is the vital ingredient, which is necessary for our survival. Walking increases your body's ability to extract oxygen from the atmosphere and distribute it to your lungs and heart and then to your blood vessels, which in turn distributes this oxygen to every cell in your body. This increased saturation of the body's cells with oxygen is also helped by the expansion (dilating) of small blood vessels, which is another direct result of walking. This blood vessel dilating process also supplies addition vital oxygen to all of your body's organs, tissues, and cells.

Walking will keep a fresh supply of oxygen coursing through your blood vessels to all of your body's hungry cells. Don't disappoint these little fellows because you depend on them as much as they depend on you. If you short-change them their daily oxygen supply, they'll take it out on you in the form of illness, disease, disability and death.

THE FIT-STEP® WALK

One of the most important things that you have to be aware of is that in order to begin a walking exercise program, you do not have to be an exercise fanatic. You don't need to engage in strenuous exercises or join a gym to engage in aerobic exercises or work-out on weight machines. It is only necessary that you do the Fit-Step Walk, which actually is just a regular daily walking program. You will see that there are many ways to augment your walking program by walking at particular times of the day or evening when you would ordinarily ride. For example, when you are driving or taking the bus to work, park or get off the bus a few blocks from your place of employment, and walk that short distance. For lunch for instance, you can take a 35 minute walk. When you're at work or at home you can concentrate on using the stairs more often. For maximum aerobic conditioning, you have to walk at least 35 minutes six days a week every week. It's really not that much exercise compared to all of the benefits that you'll accrue over the month and years that follow. The Fit-Step Walk is the most important part of any exercise program. Walking is the single most important path that you'll take towards fitness, weight-loss, good health and longevity.

Many people think that because they are active all day at home or in the office, they are getting adequate exercise. Nothing could be further from the truth. You are not expending the number of calories that are needed in a weight reduction or fitness program by these activities. There is no doubt that you are expending energy, but you will need to supplement this with your regular walking program. Most of us do not realize that we walk more than **125,000 miles in an average lifetime**, which will take us approximately five times around the entire earth. Walking is a complex physiological and biomechanical process of getting from one place to another—the act of locomotion. Walking involves hundreds of muscles, thousands of nerves, and many bones, joints, and ligaments to produce a near-perfect biomechanical method of locomotion, involving the synchronous movement of the legs and arms.

The **rhythm of walking** involves a steady pace, which will become automatic, and the brain will regulate the length of your stride, your heart rate, oxygen uptake, and other physiological adjustments. You should concentrate on making smooth, even steps, avoiding spurts of speed and abrupt changes in pace. The energy expenditure over your walking period will remain constant, and your walk should leave you feeling relaxed, with effortless motion. Colon Fletcher, author of *The Complete Walker*, said it best when referring to rhythm, "An easy, unbroken rhythm can carry you along hour after hour, almost without your being aware that you are putting one foot in front of the other."

The **speed of walking** should be approximately 3.5 miles per hour, since walking is a moderate-type exercise. If you increase the speed beyond 4 miles per hour, the upper arms and shoulders swing too fast, and the lower leg muscles have to work too hard to compensate, thus producing wasteful energy expenditure. It is important that you walk at a comfortable, brisk pace, one that does not leave you breathless. This type of walking activity falls into the **aerobic** form of exercise, in which you are taking in **oxygen** as fast as you are burning it up. This is an efficient use of energy. **Anaerobic** exercise, on the other hand, is the opposite condition, which is caused by an overexertion of muscles (e.g., running fast) working beyond their capacity. This type of anaerobic exercise leads to the buildup of **lactic acid** in the muscles, causing pain, discomfort, and fatigue, a condition known as **oxygen debt**.

The **gait of walking** refers to the motions of your legs, feet, and arms during the phases of walking. Most of the energy required for walking is provided by the muscles and joints of the ankles, knees, and hips. When we over-stride or under-stride, we disrupt the natural walking gait. An easy, steady, unbroken stride will produce the rhythm and gait necessary for the effortless act of walking. Also, it is necessary to avoid toeing in or out during the walking gait, since this wastes energy. Try to concentrate on keeping your toes straight, and thus your stride will be even and rhythmic. During the act of walking, your arms swing naturally from the shoulders. Over-swinging the arms purposely during walking will reduce the efficiency of the act of walking and subsequently tire you out early during your walk. If you don't try to concentrate on the act of walking during your rhythmic stride, you will actually allow the muscles to relax and perform more efficiently.

How About A Walk Just For Fun!

Walk whenever you can, instead of driving. If you have to drive, park somewhere a few blocks from your destination and walk the difference. Take the stairs instead of the elevator whenever possible. Take a walk when you are in a new part of town. Always walk when you are away from home to see the beauty of different surroundings. Enjoy your walk by exploring different areas around your home or office, and don't forget to look at the flowers. Take the time to smell the roses, just make sure there are no bees on them. If the weather is bad you can go to an enclosed shopping mall and walk. You can stop and look in all the windows after you've completed your regular 35-minute workout walk in the mall.

You don't have to time your pulse. You don't have to do warm up with stretching exercises before you walk. You don't have to do cool down exercises when you finish. You don't have to tire yourself or get overheated or out of breath. You don't need special clothing or equipment, just a good pair of comfortable walking shoes. You don't have to be an athlete or an acrobat. All you have to do is walk your feet for fun and you automatically, without trying, will stay fit and trim.

How Not to Have Fun!

Thousands of people who have joined fitness clubs in the past have been brainwashed by their so-called fitness instructors into believing the **"no pain, no gain" fallacy**. They have been intimidated into exercising "until it hurts," or when, at the point of total exhaustion, the instructor says, "Give me five more good ones." And if you want to look fit and trim like the twenty-one-year-old robotic fitness instructor, you'd better "use it or lose it." Most of these so-called fitness instructors have had very little or no training in exercise physiology, and very few, if any, have been certified or accredited by the American College of Sports Medicine.

In a recent survey of over 1500 women and men who participated in aerobic classes, over 53% sustained injuries. These injuries included strained muscles, sprained ligaments, torn cartilages, dislocated joints, stress fractures, and even slipped discs. Several cases of stress-induced strokes and heart attacks were included in this list of injuries. These injuries were sustained during strenuous aerobic exercises and calisthenics, and even low-impact aerobic exercises. Most people who engage in these exercises were not sufficiently conditioned to take the excessive strain put on their ligaments, muscles and joints. Once these injuries were sustained, the re-injury rate almost doubled because of inadequate healing time given for recovery in most cases.

Have You Ever Seen a Runner Smile?

Have you ever seen a runner smile? Of course not! It hurts too much. Runners hit the ground and impact their joints with approximately three to four times their body weight, so it is not unusual that over 60% of runners develop some form of arthritis by the time they're 35 to 45 years of age. The list of potential serious injuries sustained by running and other strenuous exercises include musculo-skeletal injuries, including sprains, fractures and dislocations; compressed nerves from slipped discs and various nerve injuries; bladder and kidney injuries; menstrual irregularities and uterine and ovarian damage; heartbeat irregularities, including high blood pressure, and rarely heart attacks and strokes; exercise-induced asthma, wheezing, and partial lung collapse; stress ulcers and colon abnormalities; blood-sugar abnormalities and loss of blood minerals (calcium and potassium); heat-exhaustion and heat-stroke; decreased sex-drive and infertility; retinal detachments and eye hemorrhages; anemia and other blood abnormalities; and finally, anxiety, depression and obsessive-compulsive behavior (running mania). *It certainly doesn't sound like they're having fun, does it?*

Walking is kinder to your body and produces better health, fitness and weight-control benefits than jogging or other strenuous exercises without the stress, pain and strain on your body. Medical research has proven again and again that exercise does not have to be painful in order to have beneficial results. The so-called "no pain-no gain" theory is actually insane. Walking is the only exercise that you can safely continue for the rest of your life for a healthier, happier you. *Walking certainly is the road to fitness and fun.*

WALK DON'T RUN

There is considerable agreement among most exercise physiologists that exercise on a moderate, steady basis has a tranquilizing effect. A rhythmic exercise like walking for 35 minutes seems to be the most effective method for producing this tranquilizing effect. Several theories have been proposed to explain this. One current theory is that a slight increase in body temperature affects the brainstem and results in a rhythmic electrical activity in the cortex of the brain. This produces a more relaxed state and is the direct result of exercise. Other studies indicate that there is an increase in brain chemicals, particularly a group of chemicals called the endorphins. These appear to have a tranquilizing or sedative effect and result in relaxation.

In a recent study reported in the *New England Journal of Medicine*, researchers suggested that regular exercise may increase the secretion of two chemicals called *beta-endorphin* and *beta-lipotropin.* These substances act as chemical painkillers or tranquilizers and thus can influence the body's metabolism and give a sense of tranquility and well being. This study noted that with exercise, these levels of chemicals increased, and with more strenuous exercise, this increase was even greater. This may, in part, explain the "runners' high" or the feeling of euphoria that is reported with high-intensity exercise. They stated that this also might explain the frequency with which runners sustain fractured bones while running without feeling any pain.

Walking, on the other hand, produces only a moderate rise in these brain chemicals. This results in a relaxed state of mind and produces a tranquilizing effect on the entire nervous system. Since walking is not a strenuous exercise, the level of these brain chemicals does not go too high, thus avoiding the analgesic or painkilling effect produced with high-intensity exercises. This enables the walker to be aware of pain if she or he turns an ankle or foot while walking. The runner, on the other hand, because of the high analgesic levels of these brain chemicals, may not actually feel the chest pain from a heart attack and he/she may actually drop over dead before becoming aware of the pain. The abnormally high levels of these brain chemicals in this case are another example of too much of a good thing—*the devil's deadly draught.*

The mystery of walking is just the clue you need to fight the devil's sorcery and the voodoo of everyday stress and tension. The calm, serene enchantment of walking (moderate levels of the tranquilizing brain chemicals) fights off the black arts of tension, nervousness, anxiety and stress. Let the wonderful wizard of walking lead you down the peaceful path of restful relaxation.

"No Pain – No Gain"—Not True!

I've been telling my patients and readers for the past 20 years "that moderate exercise promotes cardiovascular fitness and helps to prevent heart disease." Now a recent study reported from the Institute for Aerobics Research in Dallas proved that exercise doesn't have to be strenuous to be beneficial. In fact, they stated as their major finding that, "Just a little bit of exercise is all that is needed to lower your risk of heart disease." Additional research at the Disease Control Center in Atlanta also reported that, "Walking was as effective as any other type of exercise in preventing heart disease, without the risk of injury or disability that occurred with strenuous exercises." They further stated that, "Over 60% of adults in the United States, get little or no exercise at all." I've always contended that exercise doesn't have to be stressful, painful or exhausting in order for it to be beneficial. In my books and in my medical practice I've always refuted the exercise enthusiasts who followed the *"no pain—no gain"* myth with reference to cardiovascular fitness. Strenuous exercise programs are actually less effective than moderate walking at 3.5 miles/hr in order to develop cardiovascular fitness and good health. And it is well documented that strenuous exercises are more likely to cause muscle, bone and ligament injuries, aggravate high blood pressure, contribute to abnormal heart rhythms and have been known to rarely cause heart attacks and strokes in people with pre-existing heart or vascular conditions.

In this same study from the Disease Control Center in Atlanta, which in fact reviewed over forty previous studies on heart disease, it was also reported that a lack of exercise by itself, is as strong a risk factor for heart disease as is smoking, high blood pressure, or high blood fats. They further stated that the one statistically significant, predisposing factor in the development of heart disease which appeared in every one of the 40 plus studies, was a lack of exercise, And the exercise that they cited as the most beneficial and least dangerous, was a regular exercise walking program. Their research revealed that people who exercised the least had almost twice the risk of developing heart disease as those who exercised regularly.

It is a proven fact is that strenuous exercise is not only hazardous, but it is counter-productive to cardiovascular fitness and good health. Strenuous, short bursts of exercise contribute nothing towards the prevention of heart disease and strokes, and in fact, strenuous exercise may actually cause a heart attack or a stroke! These potentially serious consequences may be the result of strenuous exercises raising the blood pressure to dangerous levels or by causing the heart to beat irregularly (cardiac arrhythmias). I've also stated over and over again to my patients and in my books that the *"mythical target heart-rate zone"* is just that—a myth! No one has even proved scientifically that a rapid heart rate is essential for cardiovascular fitness. In fact, it could be extremely dangerous to keep the heart beating rapidly for a long period of time, especially in individuals who have undiagnosed pre-existing heart disease. A moderate increase in your heart rate is all that is necessary to achieve maximum cardiovascular fitness.

The following findings were presented by the American Heart Association:

- Despite blood pressure, cholesterol or age, moderate exercise has an independent effect in preventing heart disease and strokes.
- Men in the lower 20% of physical fitness had a 50% higher incidence for heart disease than men in the 40-60% range of fitness development.
- Women in the bottom 20% zone of fitness had a 70% higher incidence of heart disease than those women in the 30-50% range of fitness development.
- The major conclusion was that "**just a little bit more exercise**" is all that is needed to lower your risk of cardiovascular diseases, especially in women. And I think it is a bit ironic that the report ended with my long standing quotation: *"You don't need to run a marathon in order to reduce your risk of heart disease."*

WALKING AROUND KEEPS BLOOD SUGAR DOWN

Walking enables Type I diabetics (insulin dependent), to reduce their insulin requirements by approximately 35%, and Type II diabetics (non-insulin dependent) to reduce their oral medication dosages by approximately 50-75% and in some cases to eliminate medication entirely. This occurs because walking not only burns calories including sugar, but walking increases the cells' sensitivity to insulin. Type I diabetics therefore need less injections of insulin and Type II diabetics become more sensitive to the production of their own body's insulin and require less oral medication.

Once the insulin or oral medication doses are reduced, the diabetic's cardiovascular risk factors improve. A diabetic normally has increased risk factors for heart attacks and strokes. Walking appears to reduce these risk factors by controlling blood sugar, decreasing serum cholesterol, making the blood less likely to clot, reducing total body weight and by opening the tiny capillaries that feed blood to the extremities, organs, tissues, cells and to the heart muscle itself. An exercise program for the diabetic requires careful medical supervision.

All patients should get complete physical exams before starting any exercise program. For most diabetics, that means complete blood-testing, urinalysis, chest X-ray, EKG, and in some cases, a stress EKG. The patient's physician will actually determine what types of tests are necessary. Medication dosages (insulin or pills) should never be changed without a physician's approval.

In general, strenuous exercise should be avoided because it may accelerate sugar absorption which could result in sudden hypoglycemia (low blood sugar) which could result in fainting spells or other serious complications. This is particularly true if a diabetic attempts to exercise too soon after a meal. At least 60-90 minutes should elapse before a diabetic begins exercising. The beauty of a walking program is that it is a moderate aerobic-type of exercise without any of the hazards of strenuous exercise. This is especially important in the diabetic, since they are particularly vulnerable to the side effects of strenuous exercise.

Walking avoids the sudden drops in blood sugar that so often accompany strenuous exercise. Walking eliminates the high-impact stress on the extremities' nerve-endings and blood vessels, which are particularly subject in the diabetic to injury from high-impact sports. Walking gently burns calories thus lowering blood sugar moderately. This enables the diabetic to eventually lower their dosage of insulin or oral medication, after the body gradually adjusts to the wonderful world of walking. *Walking keeps your feet on the ground and your blood sugar down.*

WALK AWAY FROM TYPE A

Emotional stress can precipitate heart attacks in individuals with no known history of coronary artery disease. Type A behavior (high-strung, aggressive personalities) has also been associated with an increased incidence of coronary heart disease, completely independent of other coronary risk factors. And patients who already had coronary heart disease with Type A behavior were shown to have more severe artery involvement than did patients with heart disease who had Type B behavior (non-aggressive, more relaxed type personalities). In today's corporate America, fast paced executives with Type A personalities can be found just as often in women as in men. By climbing the corporate ladder, women and men have also climbed into a high-risk category for strokes and heart attacks. Women also have the added stress of juggling work and home responsibilities.

New research has demonstrated that emotional stress can cause coronary disease as well as aggravate it in patients who already have heart disease. And all of these studies also show that by reducing stress, coronary heart disease and hypertension can often be prevented in normal patients and controlled in patients who already have heart or blood pressure problems. Type A behavior can be modified with stress management techniques. These techniques include personal counseling, avoiding stressful situations, and our true-blue, loyal friend—*walking*. Walking has been proven over and over again to significantly reduce stress and tension, alleviate anger and hostility, decrease fatigue and malaise, and control anxiety and depression. **Walk away from stress today and your heart will be O.K.**

Turn Off the Mystery Machine

Why do we always feel as if we need to take a trip or change our environment when we're fatigued or stressed? Why do we say "Let's go to the beach" or "Let's take a trip to the mountains?" Why is it that after a hard week at the office, you feel like "just getting away from it all?" In other words, why don't we just stay put or stand still? What makes us want to get up and go? What inner force is responsible for this feeling that we must seek solace in the great outdoors, someplace away from our present confining environment?

All we know is that when a certain amount of tension builds up in our bodies we have to release it. "We've got to get out of the house." "We've got to get away from the office." "We just have to get away for the weekend." "We must get out and take a walk." Our bodies are screaming at us to release the tension. These so-called electromagnetic impulses are telling our nervous systems to shut-down the terminals. Stress is beginning to short-out our bodies like a faulty fuse. The *synapses* (connecting points) in our brains are becoming inundated with messages of stress and tension. The *neurons* (nerves in the brain and spinal cord) become overloaded like telephone wires with too many calls coming in at the same time. Whether we call this burn-out, or overload syndrome or just high-anxiety, the message is clear. Our bodies are telling us something. The message is loud and clear, like an SOS from a sinking ship. "Unplug yourself from the electric current, and turn off the mystery machine with the computer screen."

You will notice how much better you feel almost immediately after your walk. Refreshed, relaxed and relieved, you'll be better able to return to the stresses of everyday living with a new perspective on life. You will actually have built-up a type of immunity to the tensions that formerly tore you apart. This immunity, like the immunity to certain diseases, needs to be reinforced. Walking the Fit-Step way, will keep stress at bay.

WALK AWAY FROM HIGH BLOOD PRESSURE

According to the American Heart Association, over one out of every four people in the United States has high blood pressure and the incidence is higher in women than it is in men. Among people age 65 years and older, approximately two out of three people suffer from hypertension. There are approximately 57.7 million Americans who have high blood pressure according to the Heart Association Council for High Blood Pressure Research. Many of these people are at considerable risk for developing strokes, heart attacks, heart failure and kidney disease, unless they receive medical treatment. Women are particularly vulnerable to the complications of hypertension. Unfortunately, most people with high blood pressure have no symptoms; they may have hypertension for many years before it is diagnosed. Remember, always get your blood pressure checked regularly.

Many cases of mild hypertension can be controlled without the use of medication. These methods include weight reduction, salt restriction, cessation of smoking, alcohol restriction, decreasing saturated fats and cholesterol in the diet, stress reduction and exercise. It should be pointed out that the majority of studies on the benefits of exercise for lowering blood pressure have used *walking* as the best moderate intensity exercise for this purpose. Jogging and other strenuous exercises can actually raise blood pressure during the actual exercise.

Two major studies reported in a recent issue of the *Journal of the American Medical Association* proved without a doubt that regular exercise, particularly walking, can decrease the risk of developing heart disease and high blood pressure by more than 50 percent. The first report studied over 6,000 women and men who had no previous history of high blood pressure. Over a period of 4 years, people who did not exercise regularly ran a 52 percent higher risk of developing hypertension. The second study followed 17,000 women and men over a period of 16 years. Those who exercised regularly experienced only one-half the death rate from heart disease and hypertension. This study showed lower blood pressures and lower death rates, particularly in individuals who walked regularly.

In no fewer than five other separate studies in hypertensive men and women, a walking program produced lowered blood pressure in over 80% of these patients. The periods of exercise training varied in these different studies from three months to three years. It was interesting to note also, that if any individuals dropped out of the program, their blood pressure gradually went up to its former hypertensive level after six to eight weeks. This confirmed the theory that in order for exercise to be beneficial, particularly for high blood pressure, it must be carried on for a lifetime. And what better exercise than walking can be done for the rest of your life?

There are several physiological mechanisms responsible for the blood pressure lowering effect of exercise. They include improved cardiac output of blood, decreased peripheral vascular resistance to the flow of blood, slower pulse rate, dilation of small arteries, thinning of the blood and a reduced release of *catecholamines* and *angiotensin* (the hormones that cause high blood pressure). The fact remains, however, that no matter what the physiological reasons are, walking lowers your blood pressure. All you have to remember is that if you *keep your feet on the ground, you'll keep your blood pressure down!*

Don't Stroke Out!

Strokes are the third leading cause of deaths in the United States each year. The most frequent contributing factor is high blood pressure. Approximately 65% of all strokes occur in people who never knew they had high blood pressure or in people who had hypertension but did not take their medication regularly.

High blood pressure speeds up the process of atherosclerosis ("hardening of the arteries"). Untreated hypertension damages the lining walls of the arteries and allows fatty deposits to collect in the arteries. This in turn sets the stage for blood clots to form in the blood vessels of the brain, which can cause a stroke. High blood pressure also can weaken the walls of the blood vessels so that a balloon or aneurysm forms. The combination of high blood pressure and extreme physical exertion (example: jogging, weight-lifting, etc.) may cause this aneurysm to rupture, which results in a hemorrhage into the brain, producing another form of stroke.

Fortunately, stroke-related deaths have declined by almost 45% in the United States in the past 10 years. This is due primarily to the widespread, successful treatment of high blood pressure. People are realizing that they have to continue taking their high blood pressure medicine indefinitely in order to prevent strokes.

Stopping smoking also is important in preventing strokes. The carbon monoxide from smoking damages the blood vessel walls, and speeds up the process of atherosclerosis. Early treatment of diabetes and obesity also helps to slow this process of hardening of the arteries, which leads to hypertension and stroke. Also reducing salt (less than 2,400 mg daily) and stress helps lower blood pressure, which reduces your risk of stroke.

According to most medical authorities, a moderate program of regular exercise is extremely important in controlling high blood pressure and in preventing strokes. You heard it—**moderate exercise!** Walking is the exercise most often prescribed by physicians to control hypertension. Walking lowers the blood pressure and can help to prevent strokes.

Exercise and Brain Power

Women who walk regularly are less likely to experience memory loss and other brain function declines that can be associated with aging. These findings were presented at a meeting of the American Academy of Neurology. This research entailed the study of approximately 6000 women ages 65 and older. All of these women were given cognitive function testing at the beginning of the study and again after eight years. Women who walked the most demonstrated less memory loss than those in the lower exercise groups, even after adjusting for age and other coexisting medical conditions.

Researchers feel that there is a significant correlation between physical activity and chemical activity in the brain. Exercise has the ability to increase the availability of certain brain neurotransmitters (serotonin) and mood-elevating brain chemicals (beta-endorphins). There can be little doubt then, that women who walk regularly have better brain function as they age.

In a recent study in the *Annals of Internal Medicine*, it was reported that regular exercise may also delay the onset of dementia. This study showed that a moderate amount of exercise could in fact reduce a person's risk of dementia by almost 40%. Over a six year period, 1,750 adults aged 65 and older without cognitive impairment, were included in this study. The participants reported their exercise patterns at two year intervals, which included either walking, swimming, hiking, calisthenics, water aerobics, stretching, weight training, or a combination of one or more of these activities.

This study stated that the current recommendations for all adults including the elderly, should include at least 30 minutes daily of a moderate-intensity exercise to promote good health and to decrease the risk for chronic diseases and early death. They further point out that these exercise recommendations may help to prevent cognitive decline and neurodegenerative diseases in the elderly.

Walking, which is by far the best moderate aerobic exercise, combined with strength training, weight-bearing exercises, appears to be the best combination for improving physical fitness and preventing senile dementia and/or Alzheimer's disease. Swimming and water aerobics are also good alternatives or additions to your Fit-Step walking program, for a successful exercise program.

WALK OFF WEIGHT & DEPRESSION

According to a recent study, overweight women who stayed at home had a significant increase in the incidence of depression. It was further found that both obesity and depression can be alleviated by participating in a regular walking program. This study found that overweight women ages 25-40 who stayed at home experienced significantly more depression than their peers who work outside the home, possibly secondary to the lack of socialization and/or intellectual stimulation. These findings are in agreement with several other studies that have shown a positive association between exercise and mood.

The women in this study were considered moderately to severely overweight. They all exhibited complaints of mild to moderate depression. The women were randomized into a walking group and a control group who did not walk. The walking group walked 35 minutes daily, five days per week, for a period of 12 weeks. The control group did not engage in any physical exercise program whatsoever. Compared to the control group, the women who walked regularly lost weight and felt less depressed.

The results confirm studies that physical exercise, especially a moderate walking program, is a plausible treatment for mild to moderate depression, particularly in overweight women, who were stay-at-home mothers or whose jobs involved at-home duties. This walking program can act as an alternative to medication in women who prefer non-pharmacological treatment for depression, or as an adjunct to antidepressant medication. The fact that these women lost weight was a significant factor in improving the level of depression.

Walking, as we have seen, improves mood and has a natural antidepressant and a natural appetite-suppressant effect by increasing the brain's endorphins and by decreasing the brain's appetite mechanism (the appestat). A regular walking program also produces a continuous infusion of oxygen to the body's cells and also rids the body of toxins, particularly free radicals, which tend to cause degenerative changes in the body. These free radicals can not only physically alter the brain cells and cause depression, they can also cause the appetite-suppressing mechanism in the brain to be faulty and increase the level of hunger, causing obesity.

Walking women, by and large, are less depressed and less overweight, whether they are stay-at-home moms, working stay-at-home jobs, or even women who work outside the home. Walking women win the fight against obesity and depression.

EXERCISE AND ARTERIES

A study at the University of Pennsylvania showed increased blood flow into the body's arteries in patients who exercised regularly. This was apparently due to the fact that the exercise helped to keep the arteries open by decreasing the amount of inflammation inside the walls of the arteries. This inflammatory process which occurs in your arteries is a natural process of aging. The inflammation which occurs in your arteries causes the blood vessels to swell, depositing cholesterol plaques on the artery walls which in turn narrows the opening through which your blood flows. This decreased blood flow can be the cause of a heart attack, stroke or blood clot.

Moderate exercise like walking helps to keep the arteries opened by decreasing the amount of inflammation inside the walls of the blood vessels. In fact, it has been shown in repeated studies that moderate exercise helps to reduce the inflammatory process in the arteries significantly more than strenuous exercise which can in itself cause more inflammation in your body's arteries.

A Daily Walk Keeps Arthritis Away

Recent research suggests that walking may be the best exercise for most forms of arthritis. Most people with arthritis can benefit from a regular exercise program according to the majority of rheumatologists. And the exercise that most of the doctors recommended for their patients with arthritis was walking. Walking strengthens the muscles and ligaments that are attached to the arthritic joints. This helps to relieve the pain that occurs when the bones rub against each other. Walking also may prevent some of the joint inflammation and deformity that is associated with arthritis. The gentle joint motions of walking may relieve joint pain and swelling. Just make sure that you take it easy and rest frequently. Don't walk through pain.

The recurrent pain and joint swelling associated with arthritis acts as a depressant in the majority of patients with arthritis. Depression in turn leads to lethargy and inactivity. The inactivity instead of relieving the pain in most arthritics tends to lead to more joint involvement and greater immobility. Walking on the other hand with its biochemical and psychological mood-elevating effects, acts as a natural antidepressant in the arthritic patient. Walking does wonders to improve the arthritic's feeling of well-being and it improves the vicious cycle of pain, depression and subsequent immobility.

Inflammation can make the joints swell in patients who have arthritis. Doctors often give cortisone to patients with arthritis to reduce the amount of inflammation in the joints. Exercise acts like cortisone by helping to decrease the inflammation that occurs in the arthritic patient's joints. Any patient who has some form of arthritis must be monitored closely by their personal physician. Each patient is an individual and will respond differently to various forms of exercise. Just as complete inactivity may lead to a worsening of arthritis, too much activity, especially strenuous exercises, may also have an adverse effect on arthritis. Listen to the advice of your own physician.

WALKING AND COLON CANCER

A recent study at the State University of New York in Buffalo has now linked even colon cancer to a lack of physical activity. This condition had been previously thought to be caused only by a *low-fiber, high-fat diet*. Now, however, it appears that men with sedentary jobs are 60 percent more likely to get cancer of the colon compared to more physically active men.

In this study, the occupations of approximately 500 rectal and colon cancer patients were compared to the occupations of over 1,400 patients with other diseases. Women who had spent more that 20 years in completely sedentary jobs had twice the incidence of colon cancer as compared to those women with active jobs. And women who worked at low-activity jobs had 1½ times the risk of colon cancer as active workers.

Physical activity, especially a regular *walking program,* appears to stimulate the movement of waste products through the colon, thus decreasing the time that the potential waste carcinogens are in contact with the wall of the colon. This is a similar theory to that which explains why a high-fiber, low-fat diet also helps to reduce the incidence of colon cancer.

EXERCISE DECREASES RISK OF BREAST & UTERINE CANCER

In a study from Harvard School of Public Health, it was found that women who began exercising and playing sports as young girls appear to develop body changes that reduce their risk of developing breast and uterine cancers. These findings were based on the fact that exercise in young girls delays the onset of menstruation by several years. The early onset of menstruation is considered to be a potential risk factor for developing breast and uterine cancers. Active young women who engaged in sports were also noted to have fewer and lighter menstrual periods, which usually reduces the production of female hormones. This fact may be responsible for the decreased risk of developing both breast and uterine cancers in active young women.

Women who continue their exercise program into later life have less body fat and more lean muscle mass. These women also tend to eat a low-fat diet throughout their adult years. It is a known fact that excess saturated fat in the diet produces excess amounts of estrogen, which increases the risk of breast cancer. In this particular study of over 5000 women, it was also found that the leaner active women produced not only less estrogen, but a less potent form of estrogen than did inactive obese women. This less potent form of estrogen was less likely to cause breast and uterine cancer as was the more potent form of estrogen produced by overweight women. These findings showed that sedentary women had a 2½ times greater risk of developing cancer of the uterus and twice the risk of developing breast cancer.

PROSTATE CANCER PATIENTS DO BETTER WITH EXERCISE

New research suggests that exercise may be a universal supplement to the treatment of prostate cancer. The authors of a report published in the January 2011 issue of the *Journal of Clinical Oncology* used a research database and tracked the health habits of 2,705 patients who were diagnosed with prostate cancer over a period of 18 years. The researchers found that all sorts of physical activity after the diagnosis was made reduced overall mortality. This finding was independent of whatever type of prostate cancer treatment that these patients had previously received for their disease.

This report showed that men who walked for 90 minutes or more per week had a 46 % lower risk of death from all causes compared with men who walked less than 90 minutes weekly. It was also found that those men who exercised vigorously for three hours or more per week had a 49% lower risk of overall mortality and a 61% lower risk of dying from prostate cancer, compared with men who had exercised for less than one hour per week. This report also showed that men who had exercised both before and after their diagnosis was made did even better than those men who had only started exercising after they were diagnosed with prostate cancer.

FITNESS IN ADOLESCENTS AND YOUNG ADULTS

In a recent article in the *Journal of the American Medical Association*, it was shown that both adolescents and young adults with poor cardio-respiratory fitness were both at considerable risk for developing cardiovascular disease. There is strong evidence that a low level of physical activity is associated with a higher morbidity and mortality from all causes including cardiovascular disease and cancer. Population studies show that physical activity levels are extremely low in the United States, particularly in adolescents and young adults.

This study showed that adolescents and young adults with low levels of fitness were two to four times more likely to be overweight than were participants who exercised regularly. Both adolescents and young adults who were less fit were more likely to have high blood pressure and high cholesterol. There was also shown to be a relationship between low fitness levels and the incidence of the "metabolic syndrome," which consists of a combination of high blood pressure, high blood fats, obesity, and diabetes or insulin intolerance.

This report indicated that the low fitness levels in both adolescents and young adults are an important and prevalent public health problem in the United States. This correlation between low fitness levels and cardiovascular risk gives rise to a potential trend of increasing mortality and morbidity from chronic diseases caused by obesity and inactivity.

Although adolescents are not usually considered at short-term risk for developing cardiovascular disease, they do in fact develop risk factors during adolescence and young adulthood, which sets the stage for heart disease in middle and older age. There appears to be no doubt that a large segment of adolescents who are unfit and overweight are at considerable risk for developing cardiovascular disease as they age. Numerous studies in adult men and women report an association between low levels of physical activity and increased mortality from cardiovascular disease and other disorders including cancer.

It has been further shown that a regular exercise program started at any age will improve fitness and will lower the risk of developing cardiovascular disease and other degenerative diseases of aging. In order to prevent this epidemic of obesity and inactivity in adolescents and young adults from occurring, an education campaign needs to be implemented in the schools and in the work place in order to reverse these negative health behaviors. These individuals need to be educated as to the health benefits of physical activity, which is necessary to improve cardiovascular fitness and prevent this epidemic of obesity from occurring in young adults and adolescents.

THE MYSTERY OF WOMEN

"Yes, Women Are Different From Men" was the first page headline in a recent edition of *The Medical Tribune*. Finally new research has discovered that there are significant differences in the physiology of women and men. These differences extend far beyond the obvious reproductive biology differences. These differences affect almost every organ system in the body, including the heart, brain, digestive tract, nervous system and even the skin.

With reference to the heart, women's hearts beat faster at rest than do men's hearts. Also, the electrical behavior of the conducting tissue in the heart is different in women and men which may explain the normal difference in the EKG's of women and men. It has previously been found that a woman's coronary arteries are smaller than those of a man. These factors have to be taken into consideration in the diagnosis, treatment and prevention of heart disease in women. Women also present with different symptoms than men experience, when they're having a heart attack.

Physicians have to be aware of these differences when treating women with coronary artery heart disease.

Men's brains are slightly larger than women's brains; however, women's brains contain more neurons (nerve connections), which may explain why women are better at multi-tasking (juggling more things simultaneously in their lives—work, child care, home responsibilities, social activities, etc.). Women are considerably more adaptable than men, and are therefore able to cope with a variety of new situations and life changes.

A long held fallacy in medicine has been that whatever research was done on male patients, for example physiology and reactions to different medications, could be interpreted as being the same for women. Nothing could be further from the truth. For example, women metabolize various medications differently from men, which must be taken into careful consideration when treating female patients. Many diseases and medications affect women differently and therefore, these differences must be taken into consideration when formulating different types of treatments for various diseases. Yes, women are really different from men, and it's about time that the medical establishment is becoming aware of that important difference.

Many of these differences in physiology may explain the difference in the fitness response to exercise in women. The *maximum oxygen uptake* is defined as the highest rate at which oxygen can be taken up from the atmosphere and utilized by the body during exercise. It is frequently used to indicate the cardio-respiratory fitness of an individual. Even though men have a larger overall muscle mass than women, women have more long-term endurance capacity. This may in part be explained by a woman's ability to sustain her maximum oxygen uptake longer by steady, consistent exercise.

Men, on the other hand, frequently engage in short bursts of energy expenditure like jogging, racquetball, strenuous weight lifting, etc. This type of strenuous activity does not increase the maximum uptake capacity (uptake and distribution of oxygen throughout the body) for a long enough time to develop maximum aerobic fitness. Women, on the other hand, develop aerobic fitness more slowly than men; however, their fitness and endurance levels are more consistent and long lasting. In many cases, women who engage in moderate exercise activity like walking, swimming, stationary bike, treadmill, etc. are more likely to stay aerobically fit, than if they engaged in strenuous exercises. However, both men and women can achieve maximum cardiovascular fitness, weight reduction and good health on the Diet Fit-Step Plan, and get rid of those unwanted pounds.

WALKING REDUCED WOMEN'S CARDIOVASCULAR RISK

As reported recently in the *The New England Journal of Medicine*—Postmenopausal women who walk regularly, lowered their heart disease risk. This study is documented evidence that regular walking can prevent heart attacks in women. The study included over 70,000 women between the ages of 50 and 79, who were asked about the types of physical activity that they engaged in each week. None of the women included in the study had previous evidence of cardiovascular disease at the beginning of the study. During the follow-up period of 3 years, only 345 women developed heart disease.

Women who walked regularly were less likely than sedentary women to develop cardiovascular disease. Women who spent at least 2½ hours per week walking briskly were each 30% less likely than others to develop heart disease. This study also concluded that prolonged sitting appeared to counteract the benefits of any type of exercise and those women who spent more time sitting were more likely than others to develop cardiovascular disease.

WALKING SPEED PREDICTS LONGEVITY

Researchers at the University of Pittsburgh studied the walking speed and survival of more than 34,000 people, ages 65 and older, for 14 years. They found that faster walking speeds in seniors were associated with living longer. The predicted years of remaining life for each age and both sexes increased as the gait speed increased. The most significant gains were after the age of 75. This article appeared in the January 5, 2011 issue of the *Journal of American Medical Association*.

In this study, gait speed was calculated using distance in meters and seconds. All of the participants were told to walk at their usual pace. The average speed was 3 feet a second, which is about 2 miles per hour. During the course of this study, those who walked the slowest (about 1.36 miles per hour) had an increased risk of dying. Those individuals, who walked at a speed of 2.25 miles per hour, survived longer than would be expected by age or sex alone. And those people, who walked at a speed of 3 to 3.5 miles per hour, survived the longest of all of the participants studied during this 14 year period.

The researchers in this study concluded that walking is a reliable tool to measure well-being and health. Walking requires body support, power, and timing, and it places demand on the heart and lungs, the brain and spinal cord, and the bones and muscles .By the age of 80, gait speed is 10% to 20 % slower than in young adults. This study shows that walking speed is a strong predictor of survival. Walking speed may be a new sign that helps doctors separate people who are merely chronically old from those who are biologically old.

Individuals who begin the Diet Fit-Step Plan when they are younger than 65 years of age have a better than average chance of being able to continue their 3.5 miles per hour brisk walking speed as they get older. Even people who start this program after age 65 will be able to gradually build up their walking speed, providing of course that they do not have any underlying disorders. Remember that you can become physically fit at any age.

People 65 years or older, however, should have a complete physical examination first, before they attempt to increase their walking speed. Also, as I've stated previously, everyone, no matter what age, should have a complete physical examination before starting the Diet Fit-Step Plan.

Since walking is the best and most efficient aerobic exercise, it stands to reason that both men and women who continue this plan will gradually become physically fit and will have very little difficulty continuing their 35 minute walk six days per week, at 3 ½ miles per hour. On this plan these individuals will have developed maximum cardiovascular fitness and are conditioned to continue their brisk walking rate of 3.5 miles per hour. *The Diet Fit-Step Mystery Plan* is actually the fountain of youth, as this particular study points out. You will look younger, feel younger, and live longer.

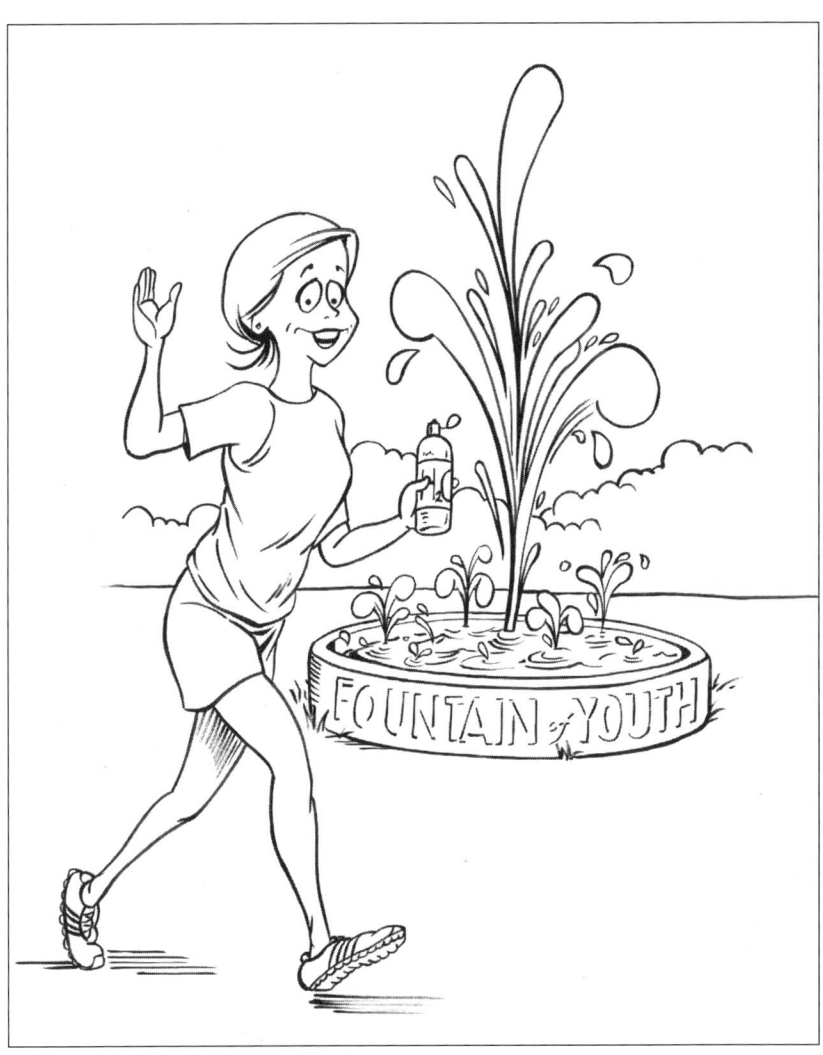

The Secret of Everlasting Youth

9

Secret of Everlasting Youth

OXYGEN: THE MYSTERY ELEMENT

Life is actually based on the six most common elements on earth, which are: carbon, oxygen, hydrogen, nitrogen, phosphorus and sulfa. Carbon is better than other elements at forming strong bonds with other carbons, linking them in chains, and adding oxygen, and the other four elements. When carbon forms long chains and large molecules it leads to the formation of wonderful things like proteins, cell membranes and DNA. Phosphorus atoms make up the important working parts of cells, including the so-called backbone of DNA, which is the part that holds the genetic code together. Phosphorous also is a critical working part of another molecule that carries the actual genetic code called RNA. In each individual cell there are strands of DNA and RNA located on particles called mitochondria, which not only contain your genetic code, but they also determine your life expectancy. The oxygen atom is critical in making all of these cells function properly and without a proper supply of oxygen these cells would slowly die.

Oxygen is the vital ingredient, which is necessary for our survival. Since oxygen can't be stored, our cells need a continuous supply in order to remain healthy. Walking increases your body's ability to extract oxygen from the air, so that increased amounts of oxygen are available for every organ, tissue and cell in the body. Walking actually increases the volume of red blood cells which carry oxygen and nutrition to the cells, and in turn remove carbon dioxide and waste products from your body's cells. This increased saturation of these cells with oxygen is also aided by the opening of small blood vessels, which is another direct result of walking. Walking every day will keep a fresh supply of oxygen surging through your blood vessels to all of your body's organs, tissues and cells. If you don't walk every day then your cells will be deprived of the essential oxygen atom that keeps the life process working. The Diet Fit-Step Plan helps to keep you looking younger and living longer, when your body is receiving its constant supply of oxygen from your daily aerobic walking program. That's the beauty of the mysterious life force called oxygen.

FEEL & LOOK YOUNGER

With the advent of the computer age, most people are forced by design to do less and less physical labor. It would seem logical that this would result in more energy being available for other activities. However, how many times have you noticed that the less you do, the more tired you feel, whereas the more active you are, the more energy you have for other activities? Exercise improves the efficiency of the lungs, the heart and the circulatory system in their ability to take in and deliver oxygen throughout the entire body. This oxygen is the catalyst which burns the fuel (food) we take in to produce energy. Consequently, the more oxygen we take in, the more energy we have for all of our activities.

Walking produces a remarkable number of changes that occur inside of your body. Your blood volume and the red blood cells increase in number. Your *heart* pumps blood more efficiently. Your lungs expand, taking in and distributing more oxygen. Your muscles tighten and contract giving you a firmer figure. Your energy level increases, and you feel strong and fit. The results of these changes will make your figure lean and your posture supreme. Your overall appearance will improve following your daily walk, since walking will improve your circulation and enable you to feel and look great. Your skin, complexion and hair texture will also improve with walking because of the increased blood circulation to the skin and hair follicles. Your complexion will literally glow after your walk and your skin will stay healthy and fresh looking all day long.

After you have been walking for a while you will notice that your muscles will become firm and many of the fatty deposits on your thighs and buttocks will start to decrease in size. Your stomach will become flatter and the muscles of your calves, thighs and buttocks will become firmer and shapelier. These changes result from improved muscle tone and also from the strengthening of muscles and ligaments, which are attached to the spine. You don't have to kill yourself to stay fit, trim and healthy. Walking actually provides better long-term figure control and fitness benefits than jogging or other strenuous exercises, without the hazards and dangers. Always remember that exercise does not have to be painful or uncomfortable to be effective. The Diet Fit-Step Plan consists of walking for 35 minutes, 6 days per week, and walking for 35 minutes using light, hand-held weights for 3 days per week, which will make you feel and look younger.

LOSE THOSE UNWANTED POUNDS

And as far as exercise is concerned, there is no doubt in anyone's mind that exercise is really a bore and most exercises usually are just too strenuous and time-consuming, Jump up, lift that, squat here, run there, or any one of a dozen useless body gyrations that leave us huffing and puffing. Or hop like a bunny on this machine or that one, so that you can exercise one tiny little muscle on each and every machine. You would essentially have to hop on a hundred different machines to exercise all of your muscle groups individually. Then you start thinking, "Did I exercise my triceps or was it my biceps?" "Was I already on that machine, or was that machine in a different row?" "To tell the truth, all of these machines look the same." "They're making me crazy; now I have to start all over again since I don't know where I began." "Maybe I should use free-weights, but what really are free weights?" All of this seems very confusing, and is easily remedied by just following the Diet Fit-Step Plan.

Studies have repeatedly shown that strenuous exercises, rather than being beneficial, are actually detrimental to our health. Strenuous exercises and lifting heavy weights can actually raise our blood pressures and make us more susceptible to irregular heart rhythms. And of course, there is all of the muscle and joint and ligament injuries that all of these over enthusiastic exercisers sustain over and over again. Won't they ever learn? I think not. People have been brainwashed into thinking that if an exercise is not painful or strenuous, then it can't be good for you. This is the so-called "no-pain no-gain myth." Nothing could be further from the truth. Medical studies have repeatedly shown that moderate exercise is far more beneficial and less detrimental to our health than those back-breaking, gut-wrenching, limb-straining types of exercises.

You don't really have to join a gym or a fitness club to exercise. You don't have to engage in lung-straining, muscle-wrenching, heart-racing, anaerobic and aerobic exercises in order to lose weight and get fit. And you do not have to subject your body to all of the torturous exercises that the so-called fitness gurus have brainwashed everyone into believing are essential for weight loss and fitness. So what do we do? Just sit there! Not really! The answer is simple. All you have to do is follow **Diet Fit-Step Mystery Plan**, which consists of an easy-to-follow diet and exercise plan that will allow you **to lose up to 15 pounds and 3 inches easily in 21 days, and lose those unwanted pounds.**

Three Easy Steps to Everlasting Youth

The Diet Fit-Step Mystery Plan is really an easy, safe and effective way to lose up to 15 pounds and 3 inches in only 21 days. You will also develop maximum cardiovascular fitness, strengthen your muscles and bones and shape your body as you follow this easy mystery program. You will actually feel and look younger and live longer on the Diet Fit-Step Plan.

1. **Step 1: The Diet-Step:35/35 Plan** simply consists of a **low-fat, high-fiber, moderate lean protein diet,** *with no more than 35 grams of fat and no less than 35 grams of fiber daily* And that's it! There are no special menus to follow, no complicated meals to prepare, and no restrictions on good tasting, nutritious healthy foods. The diet works equally well in a restaurant as it does at home. You will see from the meal plans that are included in the book, that these plans can be easily changed to meet your own individual needs and tastes. You can mix and match any number of helpful, nutritious, good tasting foods for any of your meals. You will be delighted with all of the options you have, and none of the dietary restrictions that you have been made to follow on all of those gimmick diet plans. The Diet-Step Plan is really a fun diet, and one that you can easily and safely stay on for a lifetime. Just remember to eat at least 35 grams of fiber daily and limit your total fat intake to no more than 35 grams per day.

2. **Step 2:** The second part of the Diet Fit-Step Plan is **The Fit-Step: 35 Minute Plan.** This step consists of an easy, moderate, **35 minute aerobic walking plan 6 days per week.** This walking plan can be done anytime, anywhere, or anyplace that you choose. In the morning, at lunchtime, after dinner, whenever it's convenient for you. It's your own plan. It is really quite simple. Walk at a brisk pace, approximately 3.5 miles per hour for 35 minutes, 6 days every week. Break it up into two separate walks, if your time is limited. The choice is yours.

3. **Step 3: Easy Strength-Training Exercises** combines your 35 minute daily walking aerobic exercise, along with holding one to two pound, hand-held weights as you walk 3 days per week (separated by at least one day). These weights come in several varieties. One type looks like brass knuckles turned inside out, where you just grip the padded weights with the fingers of each hand in the indentations on the weights. The other variety of hand-held weights combines a strap that goes over the back of your hand, while you hold the weights in the palms of your hand. These particular types of weights look like mini-dumbbells. The combination of walking for 35 minutes using hand-held weights is only done three days per week. This should not be done on consecutive days because it puts too much strain on the upper body muscles.

   This combination of walking using hand-held weights provides a double-blast of fat-burning calories. The reason for this is that you are burning calories by the aerobic action of walking, and you are also burning calories by the muscle-building action of the hand-held weights on your upper body. You are in a sense combining an aerobic exercise with a strength training exercise, all rolled up into one simple 35 minute walk. Sound easy? It is! And believe me; it works without any of the dangers or hazards involved in strenuous exercises or by using heavy weights for strength training and muscle building. (Chapter 10).

How Your Body Burns Calories at Rest

A new study from Yale University has shown that exercise benefits your body even at rest. Researchers studied the oxygen used by the calf muscles of the legs of both athletes and sedentary people. This use of oxygen by the muscles is known as the oxidation rate, which shows how fast muscles are burning calories while you are at rest. The researchers found that the athletes burned calories 54% faster than did sedentary people. This finding was due to the increased metabolic rate that occurred during exercise, which may help explain why the athletes were able to stay trimmer and slimmer, since they burned additional calories even while they were at rest.

The Mystery Relaxation Plan

Regular exercise can help to abate the mental and physical effects that stress has on your body. Under stressful conditions, your body responds by producing stress hormones *(adrenaline* and *cortisol),* as well as releasing fatty acids and glucose, which are used as fuel to produce energy. This combination of stress hormones and fuel products are the body's response to stress, known as *"fight or flight phenomena."* Both short-term stress situations and long-term stress conditions can lead to high blood pressure, coronary artery disease, and strokes. Also problems with digestion, headaches, anxiety, insomnia, depression, and a weakened immune system can result from long-term stress.

Physical exercise can aid the body to combat the effects of stress, by helping to burn up these stress hormones (adrenalin and cortisol) and by producing relaxing hormones called *endorphins*, which have a calming effect on the body's nervous system and help to elevate good mood feelings. Regular exercise, especially a moderate walking exercise program, helps the body combat the stress of everyday living. An aerobic exercise walking program makes you feel better and in turn helps you look better. Other relaxation activities, such as yoga and meditation, can also help you combat stress.

By combining a regular aerobic exercise walking program with strength-training exercises, using hand-held weights on the Diet Fit-Step Plan, you will actually produce more endorphins (relaxation hormones) which will help your body dissipate the stress hormones (adrenalin and cortisol). This combination is one of the best methods of dealing with stress and tension. As you continue on your Diet Fit-Step Plan, your body will continue to burn calories and increase your metabolic rate. This increased metabolic rate will boost your energy level as it decreases your stress hormones and increases your relaxation hormones. Walk away stress and tension and let the feel-good hormones wash over your body.

Power Walk Off Those Unwanted Pounds

1. Walking on **softer surfaces** like sand, dirt, or grass could help you burn an extra 100 calories in 35 minutes. This type of activity should be limited to one or two days per week.

2. **Walk up hills** as part as of your walking program on two or three days per week. This can help you burn an additional 150 calories in 35 minutes.

3. Walking on cobblestones or **uneven surfaces** uses different muscles than walking on a flat surface and burns more calories as you walk. It is important to be careful to walk carefully on these uneven surfaces to prevent ankle and/or foot strains or sprains. Also, be careful of unfortunate trips and falls.

4. Walk up and down **stairs** ten minutes every day in addition to your 35 minute walking program. This will burn an additional 100 calories per day.

5. Increase your **speed of walking** from 3.5 to 4 miles per hour for 10 minutes, and then resume walking at 3.5 miles per hour for the rest of your 35 minute walk. You can use a pedometer to calculate distance and speed of walking.

6. **Stretch your stride** so that your foot lands first on your

heel and then on your sole all the way through your stride to end up on your toes. This stretching of your stride tones and firms leg muscles and burns additional calories. Be careful not to overstretch.

7. Concentrate on **holding your tummy in** while you walk for several minutes, and then release your abdominal muscles. This burns additional calories and helps to melt belly fat.

8. **Increase your walking time** from 35 minutes daily to anywhere between 45 to 90 minutes every day. This could burn significantly more calories each day. Chapter 7—Quick Weight-Loss Walking—shows you how to lose weight more quickly by increasing the time that you walk each day. You'll easily lose those unwanted pounds more quickly.

STRENGTHEN BONES AND MUSCLES

Since the runner pounds the ground with a force equal to three to four times their body weight, she or he is more likely to sustain injuries than the walker. Walking is one of the most natural functions of the human body. Due to the structure of a person's musculoskeletal system and the shape and flexibility of the spine, the body is perfectly constructed for walking.

As you walk, the muscular and skeletal systems perform synchronously together. Your curved flexible spine has a spring-like function, made up of many vertebrae, each separated from the other by a tiny cushion (inter-vertebral disc), which is designed to absorb shock. These discs also give the spine its resilience and flexibility. When you walk, you use the hinge-like joints in your feet, ankles and knees while the ball and socket joints in your hips move effortlessly with a liquid-like motion.

The muscles that are attached to the long bones of the legs and the pelvis are specifically designed for walking. The leg, hip and back muscles are used for support and the mechanics of propelling the body forward. The long bones of the legs form a framework of levers, which are moved by these muscles, and subsequently help to propel the body forward. The abdominal muscles support the weight of the abdominal organs when you walk and your chest wall and diaphragm muscles assist in respiration.

As your legs thrust forward, you are in effect catching the forward motion of the upper part of your body. This natural motion in walking creates a perfect balance between gravity's force and the forward thrust of your body. The act of walking is therefore an almost effortless biodynamic mechanism, structurally more efficient than any woman or man-made machine. Just remember to swing your arms naturally when you walk. As you'll see in Chapter 10, the combination of walking for 35 minutes, 6 days per week using hand-held weights for three days per week, will burn more calories, and will shape and strengthen your upper body muscles. The Diet Fit-Step Strength-Training workout plan, is therefore the perfect body-shaping plan for muscle strengthening and toning, and quick weight-loss.

Flatten Your Abs with Power Breathing

A simple exercise to help tighten and flatten your abdominal muscles, is to take a deep breath and tighten your abdominal muscles. Hold your muscles taut for approximately 3-5 seconds and then release the tension as your breathe out slowly. You can do this simple exercise while sitting at your desk, watching TV, or while you're driving your car. Begin with 5 abdominal tightening repetitions 3-4 times daily, and gradually build up slowly to 10-12 repetitions every day over a 14 day period. Once you've reached 10-12 repetitions of abdominal tightening, deep breathing exercises after the first 2 weeks, then continue doing the abdominal flattening exercises every other day, in order to give your abdominal muscles time to rest between these abdominal tightening exercises. Remember, muscles need time to heal and regenerate, just like they do with any strength training, weight bearing exercises. You should space these 10-15 repetitions three to four times throughout the day. If you feel that it is too tiring, then decrease the number of repetitions until you feel comfortable.

How to Firm your Figure

The following physical and physiological effects will be noted after you have been on your walking diet for 21 days. **Muscle tone** certainly is one of the most important results we are looking for. After your daily 35 minute walk, you will notice that your muscles will be toned and firm, and after you have been on your walking program for some time, you will notice many of the fatty bulges and deposits decreasing in size. Your stomach will flatten and your calves and thighs will become trimmer, and your buttocks muscles will become more proportioned. Many of these changes are due to improved muscle tone and, secondarily, to the strengthening of the spine.

1. **Flatter stomach** – the abdominal muscles will be firm and support the intra-abdominal contents, so that the appearance will be of a flatter stomach.

2. **Slender thighs** – leg strengthening and loss of fat in the thigh muscles will reduce the outer and inner thigh dimensions.

3. **Firmer buttocks** – the large buttocks muscle, called the gluteus maximus, will contract and draw the buttocks higher and make them appear firmer.

4. **Upper arms leaner and shapelier** – the muscles of the upper arm, which include the triceps and biceps, will increase their tone, and the fat loss from the fleshy part of the upper arm will combine to form a firmer, shapelier arm.

5. **Increased level of energy** – with increased aerobic training, the lungs, heart, and circulation will be improved in efficiency and add more energy to your day.

6. **Improved nightly sleep** – a regular walking program will aid in sleep without the use of sedatives or tranquilizers.

TRIM-STEP: BEACH TONING

It is possible to almost double the number of calories that you burn when you are walking on sand rather than on hard surfaces. The reason for this is that your feet sink below the surface of the sand and your muscles, ligaments and joints have to work harder to lift your feet out of the sand. During your 35 minute walk it is possible to burn an additional 100-150 calories by just walking on sand.

Muscle toning in the areas of the calves, thighs, buttocks, and abdomen is more efficient on sand than just walking on hard surfaces. Again the reason for this is that the walking workout is more intense. Sand walking is great for beach toning which will enable you to look great in your bathing suit.

Wear a low cut walking sneaker to protect your feet from shells, rocks, glass and other beach debris. Keep your feet dry with lightweight socks to protect against blisters; however, if you are brave enough, then walking barefoot can be a lot of fun if you are careful. Don't forget to use a good sun blocker to protect your skin from the sun's ultraviolet rays. Also be careful if you have any back, knee or ankle problems because of the excess strain put on these areas by the force transmitted by sand walking, which is a high intensity type of walking. Also the uneven walking surfaces that you encounter on sand sometimes can have an adverse effect on these problem areas. Stop if you develop pain in any area of the body, and begin again after you've rested. You may tire more easily because of the increased difficulty of walking in sand. If that is the case, stop and rest and then begin again.

THE MYSTERY OF THE FIT-STEP STRETCH

Stretching exercises can improve the flexibility of the joints, muscles and tendons, thus making the body less prone to injury. Stretching also increases the flow of blood to the stretched muscle and helps to promote bone growth where there is a stretching motion against gravity. There is increasing evidence that stretching has a calming effect on the central nervous system by transmitting relaxing signals along chemical neuro-transmitter pathways from the peripheral nervous system to the brain.

Stretching should be done slowly, and stretching one muscle group at a time is preferable. For example, stretch both arms in front of you, and hold that position for 30 seconds and then let your arms down slowly, and relax them for an additional 30 seconds. Repeat this extension of both arms out to your sides, holding for 30 seconds, and then slowly letting them down and relaxing them for 30 seconds. Repeat this motion with your arms above your head, and then with your hands clasped in back of your head with your elbows bent, as if you are stretching when you get out of bed. During each of these exercises, gently stretch the arms, by actually pulling or pushing them away from the body, and then pulling them back towards the body. Remember to do it gently, and if it hurts, you're stretching your muscles too much.

Do the same procedure with your neck muscles. First look up and hold your head in that position for 30 seconds and then relax, returning to a normal head position for 30 seconds. Repeat the same procedure looking to the left, and then to the right. Also, repeat this looking down, with your chin resting on your chest for 30 seconds, and then return to the normal head position for 30 seconds. The best way to stretch your leg muscles and ligaments is to sit in a chair and stretch one leg at a time in front of you for 30 seconds, then relax the muscles, and then bend your knee, and hold that position for an additional 30 seconds, then relax the muscles and place your foot back on the floor. Repeat the same procedure with the other leg. You also can accomplish the same thing by pressing your feet into a footrest while sitting on a plane, train, bus, or at your desk.

These simple stretching exercises are designed to develop maximum flexibility of the muscles, ligaments and joints. Although not as elaborate as yoga or tai-chi, they are effective limbering and toning exercises for the body. These stretching steps help prepare the body for mental as well as physical fitness. These exercises help you to get in touch with your body as you contemplate the slow relaxing, stretching steps. Remember also to take slow deep breaths during the stretching exercises for maximum relaxing techniques. You can develop any stretching routine that feels good to you, not just those described above. Stretching is an individual exercise, and what feels good for one person may not be satisfactory to another person. Stretching can be done also by interlacing the fingers in front of your body, above your head or behind your back, while you do the simple stretching exercises described above.

Remember, if the stretching exercise hurts, either during or after the exercise, then you have stretched too vigorously. Go easy the next time. When you've finished, your muscles should feel relaxed, not taut or tight. The major advantage of the Fit-Step Stretch is that it can be done any time, anywhere or any place. When you don't have the time to walk or the weather's inclement, stretching is a viable alternative to limbering up. Stretching can also be used to warm up your muscles before your 35-minute walk.

ACTIVE OLDER ADULTS

In a study reported in the *Journal of the American Medical Association,* researchers from the National Institute of Health reported that active older adults lived considerably longer than inactive older people. This study involving over 300 older adults measured the energy expended from normal daily activities such as housecleaning, climbing the stairs, gardening, shopping, baking, and working at home or outside the home and running around after the grandkids. These individuals who expended the most energy throughout the day had a 30% lower risk of dying during the six-year period than those people who expended less energy. As I have said over and over again, it does not matter whether you join a gym, take a walk, or just do your household chores, the results are the same. You do not have to run a marathon to become fit, all you have to do is incorporate energy-expending activities into your daily routine. This study found that those adults who were the most active were those who climbed at least two flights.

THE MYSTERY WALKING CURE

People who live in areas where it's difficult to get anywhere by walking, tend to be heavier than those people who live in larger cities and towns that are less dependent on cars. It becomes apparent then that obesity is not only related to how much food people eat but it is dependent also on where they actually live. A recent study at the National Center for Smart Growth at the University of Maryland, which followed more than 200,000 Americans, found that people who lived in sprawling counties weighed an average of 6-7 pounds more than those who lived in more compact densely populated areas. In another related study, it was found that for every hour that people spend in their cars, they are 10% more likely to be obese.

Although more than 75% of all errands are less than one mile from home, walking does only 25% of these trips. Unfortunately, in some suburban areas where there are no sidewalks or where intersections and crosswalks are some distance apart, walking is not an option. The vast majority of children live within one mile of school; however, less than 25% actually walk to school. This may in part be related to safety reasons, but the fact remains clear that both adults and children, especially those living in sprawling suburban communities walk less than their city counterparts.

These studies show one important finding: the less you walk the more you weigh! So, what's the solution? Well no matter where you live, you should make a concerted effort to walk more every day. Whether it's several times around the block or several times around the mall, walking is the secret cure for obesity. Most people don't have time or money to join a health club or gym, but walking can be done anywhere, anytime and most anyplace. If you have to drive to work or to the store, park a little farther from your destination, so that you'll at least get some walking done. Whenever possible, take the stairs instead of the elevator at work or when shopping. Remember, to walk as much and as often as you can every day in order to lose weight, get physically fit and stay healthy.

Live Longer with Diet Fit-Step Plan

1. Walking lowers the blood pressure by:

    A. dilating (opening) the arteries, allowing more blood to flow through them

    B. improving elasticity of blood vessels-giving less resistance to the flow of blood

    C. lowering chemicals in blood that can raise blood pressure-catecholamines and angiotensin

    D. improving return of blood to the heart, so that the heart can work more efficiently at a slower rate

    E. increasing the amount of oxygen delivered to all tissues and cells

    F. decreasing the rate of sodium reabsorption in the kidneys

2. Walking protects the heart by:

   A. decreasing the risk of blood clot formation

   B. improving the return of blood to the heart from the leg veins

   C. increasing the flow of blood through the coronary arteries

   D. increasing HDL (good) cholesterol which protects the heart and arteries against fatty deposits (plaque)

   E. improving the efficiency of the heart's cardiac output (total volume of blood pumped out by the heart each minute)

   F. helping to keep the collateral circulation open and available for emergencies

3. Walking improves lung efficiency and breathing capacity by:

   A. conditioning the muscles of respiration (chest wall and diaphragm)

   B. opening more usable lung space (alveoli)

   C. improving efficiency of extracting oxygen from the air

4. Walking improves the general circulation by:

   A. increasing the total volume of blood, and the amount of red blood cells, allowing more oxygen to be carried in the bloodstream

   B. dilating the arteries, thus improving blood flow

   C. increasing flexibility of arteries, thus lowering blood pressure

   D. compression of leg and abdominal veins by the pumping action of the muscles used in walking, aiding the return of blood to the heart

   E. using small blood vessels in the legs for re-routing blood (collateral circulation) around blocked arteries in emergencies

5. Walking prevents the build-up of fatty deposits (plaque) in arteries by:

   A. decreasing the serum triglycerides (sugar fats)

   B. decreasing LDL (bad) cholesterol in the blood

C. increasing HDL (good) cholesterol in the blood

D. preventing the blood from getting too thick, thus lessening the chance that blood clots will form

6. Walking promotes weight loss and weight control by:

A. directly burning calories

B. regulating the brain center (appestat) to control appetite

C. re-directing blood flow away from digestive tract toward the exercising muscles thus decreasing appetite

D. using blood fats instead of sugar as a source of energy

7. Walking controls stress by:

A. increasing relaxation hormones in the brain (Beta-endorphins) and decreasing stress hormones (epinephrine and norepinephrine)

B. increasing the oxygen supply and decreasing the amount of carbon dioxide to the brain

C. efficient utilization of blood sugar in the body regulated by an improved production of insulin

D. literally walking away from stress

8. Walking promotes a longer healthier life by:

A. strengthening the heart muscle and regulating the cardiac output (a slower more efficient heart rate)

B. lowering blood pressure, thus preventing strokes, heart attacks and kidney disorders

C. improving lungs' efficiency in extracting oxygen from air

D. improving the efficiency of the delivery of oxygen to all the body's organs, tissues and cells

E. strengthening muscle fibers throughout the body thus improving reaction time and maintaining muscle tone

F. maintaining bone strength and structure by preserving the mineral content of the bone, thus preventing osteoporosis (bone thinning) and certain forms of osteoporosis

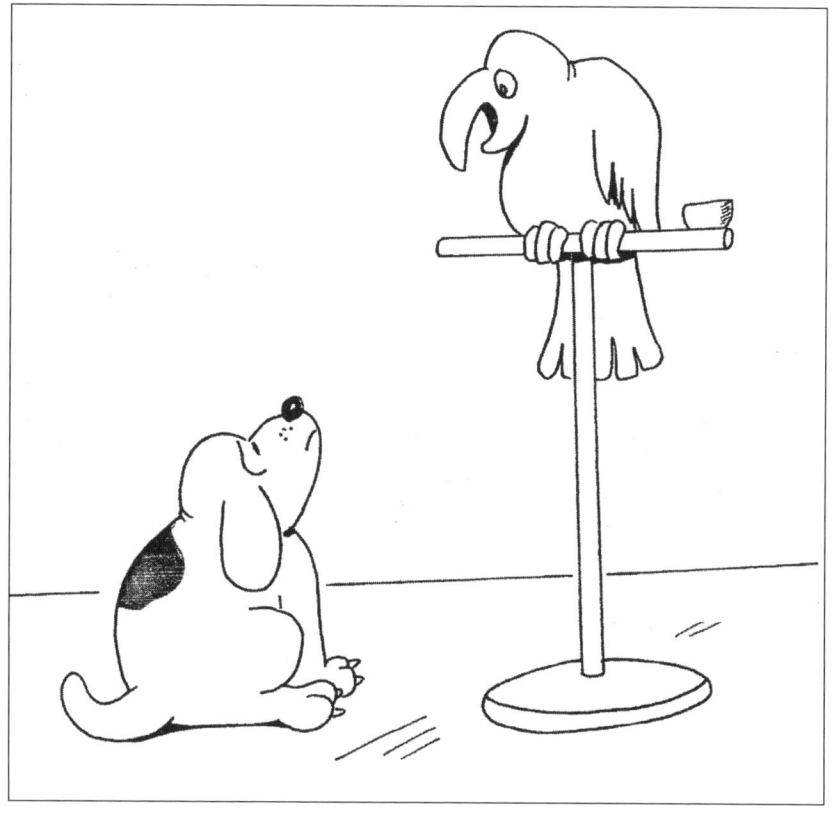

"I'm 125 years old. I think it's because I eat like a bird."

234 The Case of the Unwanted Pounds

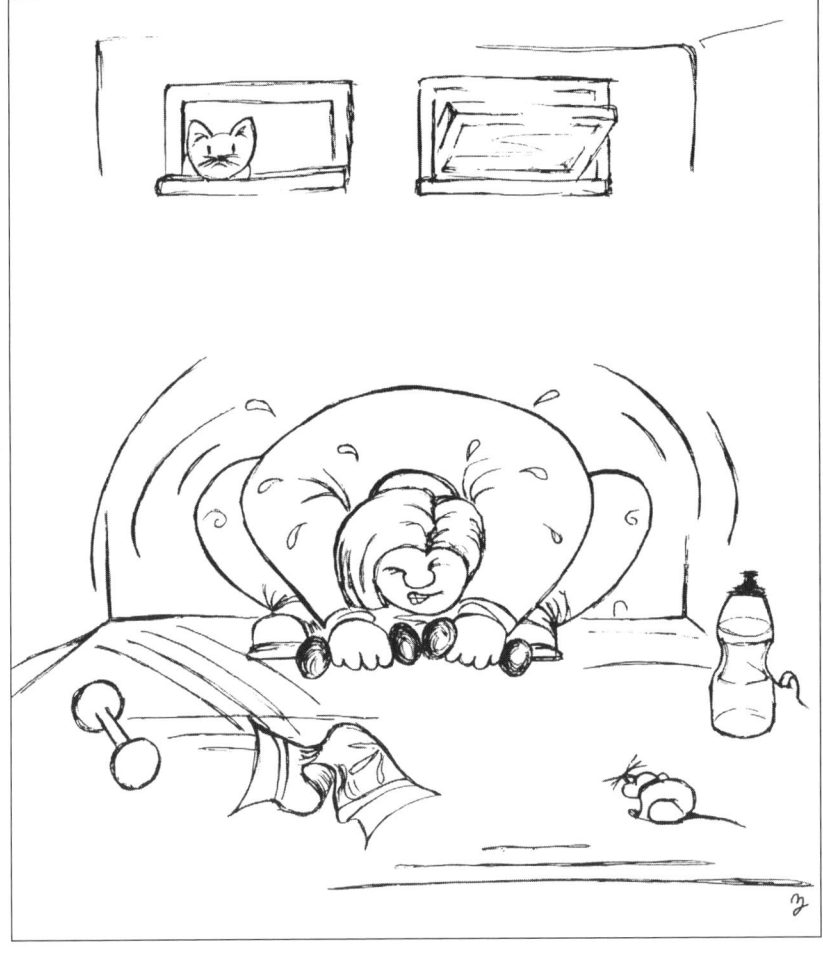

10

Body-Shaping Mystery Solved

THE MYTH OF CELLULITE

Many books, videos, tapes and health clubs promise to shape your body, improve your figure, sculpt your muscles, or get rid of cellulite. Most of these programs involve strenuous exercises, painful muscle stretching, core body strengthening, massages, or phony creams and ointments. First, real body-shaping is difficult if not impossible to achieve by any of these methods. Most individuals who want to shape their figure usually find that strenuous exercises or muscle stretching or any of these methods don't offer permanent results. Many diet books recommend low carbohydrate diets to melt belly fat, which subsequently will shape your body. However, most if not all fad diets, especially low carbohydrate diets, cause more problems than they're worth. People who follow these fad diets often develop kidney and liver problems while they're attempting to lose weight. The weight loss that initially occurs with low carbohydrate diets comes from water loss. Then the weight loss that follows usually comes from the breakdown of muscle tissue rather than from burning fat calories. The metabolism instead of burning fat for energy actually begins to store fat, in an attempt to conserve energy, because it wants to prevent the body from starving to death, which it believes is happening from the low carbohydrate diet. Once the diet is stopped, rebound weight gain occurs, and the individual gains more weight than she or he lost before starting the diet. No body-shaping for you!

Now what about those lumpy, bumpy hips and thighs? First of all, don't let anyone give you the baloney about *"cellulite deposits."* There's no such thing as cellulite! It's a term coined by diet promoters to encourage people to purchase diet-gimmicks to rid themselves of the mythical cellulose. Microscopic studies of fat show that fat cells are connected by strands of connective tissue. When these connective tissue strands stretch, they lose their elasticity and subsequently the fat takes on a lumpy appearance. Regular fat cells and the so-called cellulite fat deposits are indistinguishable under the microscope. *Fat is fat!* And cellulite is phony-baloney. You can't correct this by creams, ointments, strenuous exercises or stretching your body.

BE FIT, FIRM & STRONG

Tell most people that walking produces a flat tummy, slim hips and thighs and they'll tell you that you're crazy. "You need to do strenuous calisthenics and exercises to reduce fat deposits in those areas." Don't be too sure! Walking can give you a flat, firm tummy and slim hips and thighs without any additional exercises. However, when you also do the easy Fit-Step Walking Workout Exercises using hand-held weights, you'll quickly develop a trimmer, more sculptured figure. First, when you walk briskly with an even stride you are contracting and relaxing muscles in your chest, back and abdomen. With each forward motion of your legs, these muscles contract to keep your body erect. Your abdominal muscles tighten automatically, exactly as they would if you were doing strenuous sit-ups, and you're not straining your back muscles. As you swing your upper arms, the upper chest wall muscles that are tied in with the upper abdominal wall muscles aid in tightening these abdominal muscles.

This combination of upper body and lower abdominal muscle contractions is what produces *a firm, flat tummy*. With repeated bouts of walking, come repeated bouts of muscle tightening, until a point is reached when your abdominal muscles are firm and taut all of the time, whether you're walking or not. This firm, flat tummy will continue to last as long as you walk regularly. Also as you walk, the forward and backward motion of each hip stretches the hip muscles. This hip motion tugs at your lower abdominal muscles, further flattening your tummy.

Since walking is a moderate aerobic exercise, it burns fat rather than muscle tissue. The result: *trim hips and thin thighs*. When this aerobic walking exercise fat-burning process is combined with weight-bearing exercises (hand-held weights), you will trim down the fat deposits on those lumpy, bumpy hips and thighs. This won't get rid of the mythical cellulite, but it will give the impression of reducing its appearance, because of the strengthening of the surrounding muscles and the supporting ligament structures. Sounds too easy? It certainly is! It's the *Diet Fit-Step Easy Body Shaping Plan.*

The forward motion of your legs combined with the tightening of the lower abdominal muscles also produces a tightening effect of your lower back and buttocks muscles. This combination of alternate muscle groups contracting and relaxing produces firm, tight buttocks muscles. This firming effect actually lifts the buttocks so that they lose their saggy appearance. Your thighs will also become thin and trim and will remain that way as long as you continue your 35 minute walking program 6 days per week, while using your hand-held weights 3 days per week for strength-training

Your posture will also improve as you strengthen your shoulders and back muscles. Your head will assume an erect position and your back and spine will straighten. Your buttocks and thigh muscles will tighten and firm up, and your upper arms will lose their flabby appearance. Your figure will slowly go through a metamorphosis and you will appear younger, feel better and be healthier than you ever were before. The best, and most effective, and the easiest way to develop tight abs, trim thighs and firm buns, is to walk for 35 minutes, 6 days per week, and walk for 35 minutes using hand-held weight three days per week as described in the *Diet Fit-Step Strength-Training Exercise Plan.*

STRENGTH-TRAINING BURNS FAT

Studies reported at the 2008 Experimental Biology Meeting, showed that short, simple, weight-training workouts helped men and women of all ages lose weight and keep that weight off permanently. Weight-training also was shown to strengthen the body's immune system, as well as lower the blood pressure. By following a low-fat, moderate protein and complex carbohydrate diet, combined with simple weight-training exercises for fourteen weeks, the participants in this study lost fat deposits and weight, and increased the proportion of muscle relative to their body weight. Also, these men and women showed significant improvements in blood pressure, heart rate, and aerobic fitness.

Another similar study showed that middle-aged and elderly people developed stronger muscles and a healthier immune system while walking regularly, combined with weight-training exercises. Many of the middle-aged and elderly people in this study were moderately obese when they started the program. After twelve weeks, the majority of the obese participants had lost considerable weight, in addition to gaining lean muscle mass. These individuals also developed improved cardiovascular fitness, in addition to gaining muscle strength and boosting their energy levels.

Contrary to popular belief, you can exercise after you eat as long as you wait at least 30-45 minutes, particularly with a moderate intensity exercise program like walking. The benefits of walking immediately after eating is that it improves the digestive process, helps to resist tempting desserts, and power boosts your metabolism and burns some of those extra calories that you should not have eaten anyway. By redirecting some of the blood supply away from the digestive track, walking helps to reduce post eating drowsiness. Walking actually speeds up the digestive process called peristalsis, which moves food along the intestinal passage at a faster rate. This increase in peristalsis prevents the absorption of many unwanted fats and sugars into the bloodstream.

The basal metabolic rate—like the energizer bunny—keeps on

ticking even after you have stopped walking. Your body's normal resting basal metabolic rate burns approximately one calorie per minute (CPM). During your regular 35 minute daily walk at 3.5 miles per hour, your basal metabolic rate increases to five calories per minute. Now, here is the so-called *"slight-of-hand-walking-trick."* When you stop walking your basal metabolic rate does not return to its resting one calorie per minute rate. Your body's metabolic rate got so revved up from your 35 minute walk it continues to remain elevated for up to six hours after you have stopped walking. This increased rate will not remain at five calories per minute, but it will stay at between two to three calories per minute for the next six hours. What does all that mean? Well, if you walk for 35 minutes during lunch, when you get back to the office and are stuck behind your computer for the rest of the day, your body's metabolic rate will be burning two to three calories per minute, instead of the usual sedentary one calorie per minute if you had not walked at lunch time. The same process will occur if you take a one half hour walk after supper. You will actually be burning an additional two to three calories per minute while you are sleeping rather than the resting one calorie per minute metabolic rate. This means that you will burn more calories every day while you walk and at rest after you walk.

In effect, you have discovered a double dose of calorie burning. One with exercise and one with rest. Not too shabby. Your body is actually giving you a bonus for exercising. It is saying to you, "Well, if you are smart enough to exercise, then you deserve a bonus for your good work." Your body is a wonderful machine and it gives you a reward for using, and not abusing it. Your body is actually saying to you, "Lets work together toward good health, physical fitness, and weight loss, and if you exercise and keep your metabolism revved up, then I will keep the motor going when you stop to rest." I would say that is a unique combination that is impossible to beat.

IMPORTANCE OF STRENGH-TRAINING

A new study by the American Heart Association recommended resistance training for people with or without cardiovascular disease. It was shown that there are considerable benefits to improving muscular strength in addition to the benefits of a regular aerobic exercise walking plan. Lifting weights or exerting force against resistance is an integral part of an over-all exercise program for weight reduction and cardiovascular fitness.

Both resistance training and aerobic exercise (walking) have different positive effects on fitness development in your body.

1. Aerobic exercise (walking) has a moderate effect on the percentage of body fat; resistance training has only a small effect.
2. Resistance training has a moderate affect on lean body mass and major affects on muscular strength, while aerobic exercise has little affect on both.
3. Both aerobic exercise and resistance training produce similar beneficial effects on both the HDL and the LDL cholesterol, whereas aerobic exercise has a greater affect on lowering serum triglycerides.

Resistance training is now fairly well recognized in cardiac rehabilitation programs. People with a history of heart failure or heart disease can improve their functional capacity, physical strength, endurance, and the quality of their lives, by the addition of strength training exercises to their aerobic walking exercise program. This type of exercise, which includes strength-training exercises, especially in the elderly, must be under careful medical supervision.

YOU'RE NEVER TOO OLD TO STRENGTH TRAIN

According to the American Heart Association, strength training exercises can even help heart failure patients and nursing home residents gain strength for everyday living. In a 10 week resistance training program, elderly nursing home residents, even those with a previous history of heart attacks or heart failure, have been shown to be able to increase their strength by 43%, and their distance walked in 6 minutes by 49%. These resistance training exercises included abdominal crunches, lifting light weight dumbbells, and using hand-held weights while walking. This study recommended that elderly people begin with low levels of strength training and gradually increase the number of repetitions before adding additional weight or resistance.

This particular study, which was reported in a recent issue of the *Journal of Circulation*, stated that resistance training, whether it was doing sit-ups or lifting weights, should be used as a complement to a regular aerobic exercise program for maximum cardiovascular benefits. It is important to note, that these elderly patients must be under careful medical supervision, before, during and after performing strength-training exercises.

Aerobic exercise and weight training regularly may slow the onset of arthritis and improve joint movement. A recent study showed that people who exercise regularly had significantly less muscle and joint pain as they got older. When you add strength-training exercises to your aerobic walking program, you build stronger bones and muscles. This combination of an aerobic walking exercise program and strength-training exercises boosts calorie burning for additional weight-loss, boosts your metabolism, provides more energy and shapes and tones your body's figure.

BUILD MUSCLE MASS

Men and women after 35 to 40 years of age begin to lose muscle mass at a rate of approximately one-third pound per year. Strength training exercises make your muscles stronger and strengthen your bones. The muscles and ligaments attached to your bones create a traction or tension on the bones when you exercise. This traction causes your bones to strengthen, by helping to absorb more calcium into the bones from the bloodstream. This process increases the mineral content of the bones, thus strengthening your bones and making them less brittle, so less calcium is lost from your bones as you age.

Aerobic exercise is great for cardiovascular fitness and burning calories, but it does not build body muscle mass. Unless we exercise, fat replaces muscle as we age. The necessity for strength training is even more pronounced in women because they begin with more fat cells and less muscle tissue compared with men. Strength training is therefore essential for weight control, strong bones and muscles and overall fitness and well-being in everyone over the age of 35 to 40 years.

Many studies have shown that people who engage in strength training exercises develop an increase in skeletal muscle mass, whereas sedentary people lose considerable muscle mass over a period of time. Bone mineral density also increases by 1.5 % with strength-training and decreases by 2.5% in sedentary people. Also, studies showed that strength-training in both men and women increased their lean muscle mass by 4% and decreased their fat mass by 8%. This means that your muscles will become more shapely and defined and you will feel stronger because your muscles are actually stronger. You will have greater joint flexibility and have more energy when you walk. Your bones will be structurally stronger and, you will be less likely to develop osteoporosis or thinning of the bones as you get older.

Weight resistant exercises build your body's muscle mass. Improved muscle mass burns more calories by boosting your metabolism. When you build up your lean muscle mass, you can actually burn 35% more calories with exercise then you can if you were not doing strength training or strength resistance exercises. *Muscle cells are more efficient at burning calories than fat cells.*

On the other hand, if you just diet without exercising, you can actually lose muscle mass and subsequently decrease your basal metabolic rate. This means in effect that your basal metabolic rate slows down, so that even if you reduce your calorie intake, you will probably lose very little, if no weight at all. If you just add walking, you will increase your basal metabolic rate to five calories per minute, and if you add strength training exercises, you will increase your basal metabolic rate to six to seven calories per minute as you build muscle mass. This is the main reason that most people who do not exercise cannot lose weight, or if they do lose weight initially, they plateau and the weight remains the same. Only by using the combination of an aerobic exercise like walking and an exercise like strength training with hand-held weights, can you actually lose weight effectively and permanently. And only then can you break through the so-called impossible plateau that happens with each and every diet.

THE MYSTERY MUSCLE BUILDER

You may think that the only way to build muscle mass is to do strength or weight training exercises. Or you may think that it's necessary to consume more protein in your diet in order to build muscle mass. You're correct on both counts; however, there's another secret sure-fire way to build muscle mass which is to consume *potassium rich foods* such as bananas, cantaloupes, sweet potatoes, pumpkin, avocado, oranges, tomatoes, sweet potatoes, winter squash and apricots. All of these fruits and vegetables can be found in your local markets or produce stores.

Potassium appears to counter the effects of certain foods such as meats and refined grain cereals and breads, which create acid residues in the body that leads to muscle wasting. Fruits and vegetables, on the other hand, become alkaline in the body when digested, which in effect, neutralizes the acidity of other foods.

As we age, our muscle mass declines slowly after the age of 45. However, in a recent study, people over the age of 50 who ate lots of potassium rich foods, gained approximately 3.5 more pounds of lean tissue muscle mass than those who consumed one half as much potassium.

DOUBLE BLAST OF CALORIE BURNING

Weight resistance exercises can include weight lifting, sit-ups, push-ups, aerobic exercises, swimming with flippers, skiing with poles, or walking with hand-held weights. Of all the weight resistant exercises, walking with hand-held weights is the most efficient. That is because it combines the aerobic fitness benefits of walking with the strength training exercises of hand-held weights. You actually have a double blast of calorie burning by walking with hand-held weights. First you burn calories by the aerobic exercise of walking, and secondly, you burn additional calories by building muscles using strength training exercises. It is also the easiest type of weight training since you are not subjecting yourself to strenuous exercises or heavy weights, which can make you prone to injuries.

In addition to this double blast of calorie burning, energy boosting exercise, you get a double reward from your body. As we previously said, when you stop walking your basal metabolic rate does not decrease to the resting one calorie per minute rate. The basal metabolic rate stays at about two to three calories per minute for up to six hours after you stop walking. But now that you have added weight resistance in the form of hand-held weights to your walking program, you are actually building additional muscle mass. And as we said previously, muscle burns calories at a faster rate than fat cells and therefore you will burn additional calories after you have stopped using the hand-held weights. This means at rest, you can add another one calorie per minute burn to your walking with weights program. This translates into approximately three to four calories per minute burned when you are at rest after you have walked with hand-held weights. This means that you are almost burning as many calories resting after your walk with weights as you did when you were actually walking without weights. It sounds impossible doesn't it? Well, it's not! Have you ever noticed how fit, trim, muscular toned individuals can eat considerably more than unfit individuals. The reason for this is that they are always burning calories either during exercise or at rest.

Another way to boost your metabolic rate is to vary your walking speeds during your 35 minute walking program. Walk the first 15 minutes of your 35 minute walk at a brisk pace of approximately 3.5 miles per hour, and then speed up your walking speed to 4 to 4.5 miles per hour for approximately five minutes. Then resume walking at 3.5 miles per hour for the last 15 minutes minutes of your 35 minute walk. Here you have to be careful not to overtax yourself. If five minutes of the faster speed seems too tiring for you, then use two or three minutes of faster walking at 4 to 4.5 miles per hour. If that seems to fatigue you, then try one minute at a faster rate, for two or three times during your 35 minute walk. By increasing your speed of walking you will actually boost your basal metabolic rate to approximately six calories per minute. Do not try to fast walk every day, maybe just once or twice a week. Also, remember that by increasing your exercise basal metabolic rate to six calories per minute, your post exercise resting basal metabolic rate will be that much higher. If you find that increasing your speed is too tiring then don't do it.

Walking With Weights

I usually recommend 1-pound cushioned hand-held weights, with either straps attached that go around the back of your hands, or hand-held weights with grooves for your fingers to grip the weights. After using the 1-pound weights with walking for about four-six weeks, I advise my patients to graduate to the 2-pound weights. It is important to start with one pound hand-held weights and gradually build up to two pound weights after a four to six week period. If you find that two pound hand-held weights are too heavy, then just continue your walking with weights program using one pound weights. These weights should be cushioned and covered with rubber or vinyl, since they won't rust and aren't cold to grip in cold weather. You can also purchase comfortable held-weight that are cushioned weights with soft-foam grips, with or without secure hand straps.

A sure-fire way to boost your calorie burning workout is to

walk with hand-held weights. Using hand-held weights makes you work harder and improves your cardiovascular conditioning while building upper body strength. Always check with your doctor before walking with hand-held weights, especially if you have any medical condition. Also be especially careful if you have back or joint problems before walking with weights. If you find it causes any pain or discomfort, discontinue using weights while walking.

When you start your walking with weights program, take 5 minute walks every other day for the first 7 days, so that you don't over stretch your muscles and joints. Then build up to 10 minutes of walking with weights every other day for the next 7 days. After that, walk for 15 minutes every other day for the next 7 days. Starting at day 21, you can start your 35 minute walk with hand-held weights, three times a week. Initially, avoid any hills during your first six weeks while walking with hand-held weights to avoid over stressing or over stretching your muscles and joints.

Do not use weighted vests around your back or chest since they will throw off your center of gravity and make walking more difficult and dangerous since you will be prone to falls and back strain. Also avoid the use of ankle weights since they will cause you to strain your ankles and knees while walking. Injuries to these joints include ankle sprains and strains and ligament and tendon tears and cartilage injuries, especially to the knees. Ankle weights make walking difficult and strenuous and significantly increase the incidence of shin splints. Also, avoid wrist weights which can cause hand and wrist ligament injuries, and can actually impair your normal arm-motion swing when you walk.

Walk with a normal arm motion as you would walk without weights. Swing your arms close to your body in a short arc. Be careful not to over swing your arms as you can increase the risk of tendon, ligament and muscle injuries if the weights are swung in an exaggerated arc, especially above the shoulder areas. It is important to develop a walking stride and arm swing that is comfortable for you. Do not swing your arms at a greater speed than you would if you were walking naturally without weights. Also do not swing your arms at a slower rate than you would swing them without weights because they will create a dead load on your ligaments and joints and make them prone to injury.

Walking three times a week is all that is necessary to build upper body strength and muscle mass. Even after you walk with weights you will continue to burn calories at a faster rate than you would if you had just walked without weights. This is because your metabolism continues to burn excessive calories even after you are finished with your exercise. Walkers burn approximately 25% more calories doing the Diet Fit-Step Plan using hand-held weights. Also, walking with weights *builds lean muscle mass, which burns an additional 50 calories an hour per 1 pound of muscle.* This activity is excellent for people of all ages and helps to maintain strong rotator cuff and shoulder muscles. Walking with weights also helps to develop good muscle tone, which improves balance and stability when walking. Also, walking with hand-held weight helps you to develop good posture and strong chest and abdominal wall muscles.

These changes occur because of the combination of the fat-burning aerobic walking exercise and the strength-training, upper body muscle-building exercise, when you use hand-held weights while walking. This is a combination that is truly impossible to reproduce. You don't have to do separate aerobic and strength-training exercises at different times or on different days. It's all combined in one easy, user-friendly exercise. Walking with weight just three days per week is all that you'll need to develop cardiovascular fitness, permanent weight loss, and a figure to die for! Both men and women benefit from the Diet Fit-Step Strength-Training Exercises. These exercises are ideal in helping to prevent osteoporosis, since walking with hand-held weights puts the necessary tension on the bones and muscles, which is essential in preventing bone loss. The Diet Fit-Step Strength-Training plan of walking with weights is essential in helping to improve cardiovascular fitness, thus lowering blood pressure and also helping to reduce the incidence of heart disease and strokes.

Always check with your own physician to see if he/she feels that you are physically healthy and fit to walk with hand-held weights.

Diet Fit-Step Strength-Training

Weight resistance exercises are good for your muscles and especially good for the body's most important muscle--your heart. In a recent study by the American Heart Association, it was reported that strength training exercises can significantly lower blood pressure. Those individuals who regularly lifted light weights experienced a reduction in the systolic blood pressure (when your heart muscles contract) and a reduction in the diastolic blood pressure (when your heart muscles relax). Their resting blood pressures dropped regardless of a person's body size or weight, or whether they used heavy weight resistance exercises with longer rest periods or lighter weight exercises with shorter rest periods. In other words, using lighter weights as we suggest in the **Diet Fit-Step Walking Workout Plan,** causes the same reduction in blood pressure as those people who are lifting heavier weights. And actually lifting heavy weights can be dangerous to your health, because over the long run they can actually raise your blood pressure. Weight resistance exercises particularly using lighter weights as in the Diet Fit-Step Strength-Training Plan is safe and effective, for weight reduction and building strong bones and muscles. It's important for everyone to have a complete physical examination before using hand-held light weights, especially for individuals who have had a previous heart attack, angina, high blood pressure, and irregular heart rhythm or heart valve problems.

In another recent report released by the American Heart Association, there is now increasing evidence that strength training can favorably modify many risk factors for heart disease, including blood fats (cholesterol and triglycerides), blood pressure, body fat levels and glucose metabolism. Until recently, the conventional thinking was that strength training exercises helped to build and sculpt your muscles, but did little to help the cardiovascular system and might even be harmful to your heart. This current study dispels many of the misconceptions regarding strength training. The current study showed that strength training is beneficial using light weights for strength training.

The American Heart Association's finding in their latest study showed that weight resistance exercises should be of moderate intensity. In other words instead of the fallacy "no pain-no gain," the truth as I've always told my patients, is "train, don't strain." The Diet Fit-Step Walking Workout Plan makes your body leaner and your muscles more defined and sculptured. In addition, this plan builds stronger bones and muscles, straightens your posture, and strengthens your joints and ligaments. This plan also boosts your metabolism, which in turn helps you to lose weight. And finally, strength-training exercises enhance your sense of well-being and your self-confidence. In other words, a new vital improved you will be full of pep when you do the Diet Fit-Step.

So you will see that the Diet Fit-Step Walking Workout Plan not only makes you feel and look great, but helps to strengthen your heart and lower your blood pressure. In addition, it sculpts and molds your body into a figure supreme and a body that's lean. Not a bad combination for a 35-minute walking-workout three times a week using hand-held weights. This plan provides the unique power combination of strength training and aerobic fitness conditioning.

FIT-STEP WORKOUT CLUES

1. WALKING WORKOUT

No matter how long you walk, your upper body, particularly your arms, shoulders chest and upper abdomen, get a free ride. Walking is not enough to build upper body strength. Even if you pump your arms vigorously while you walk, your upper body does not get stronger because there is no resistance to encounter while you walk. On the Diet-Fit Step Plan however, your legs get stronger because they encounter the resistance of the ground and thus support your body's weight. In other words your legs get stronger, your thighs, buttocks and hips get firmer and your abdomen gets flatter.

Weight resistance using hand-held weights while walking is a great way to put your arms to work and to strengthen your upper body muscles. This combination of walking with hand-held weights actually makes you a stronger walker. A walker's upper body should be geared towards strength and endurance, not building muscle bulk. In other words, we want to sculpt and mold the upper body (arms, back and chest). Therefore, the key to the Fit-Step Diet walking workout plan is to use light-weight, hand-held weights while walking 3 days per week, while you continue your 35 minute walking plan for 6 days every week.. Remember, never to walk with weighs on consecutive days, because of the possibility of injury to your muscle fibers. These fibers need at least 24-36 hours to regenerate themselves, before muscle strength-training exercises.

2. WILL WEIGHT TRAINING MAKE YOUR MUSCLES BULK-UP?

Many women have the misconception that weight training will result in building ugly massive muscles. Nothing could be further from the truth. In reality, women don't have to fear developing bulky muscles because of the increase in basal metabolic rate which occurs during the Diet Fit-Step strength training exercises. Since muscle actually burns more calories than fat; your muscles become more defined, as your muscle tissue replaces fat cells. Since women have more body fat than men, they are less likely to bulk up like men who have more muscle mass to begin with. Women will see improvement in muscle tone and strength after only 21 days on the Fit-Step strength training exercises. Muscles will become more defined and sculptured for a trim, firm look in both men and women. Remember this is not strenuous heavy weight lifting, this is a walking workout with light-weight, hand-held weights.

3. HOW THE FIT-STEP HELPS YOU LOSE WEIGHT

As you walk with light-weight, hand-held weights, you build muscle mass, which in turn speeds up your metabolism. Muscle tissue burns more calories than fat cells burn; therefore, building muscle helps boost your resting metabolism. This increase in the resting metabolism occurs because of the actual increased muscle mass that you develop and the increased metabolic activity in the muscles themselves. By combining your 35 minutes of aerobic walking (Fit-Step) with strength-training exercises using hand-held weights (Diet Fit-Step Strength-Training), you have the advantage of a "power blast" of calorie burning for weight loss, while you're firming and toning your body's muscle mass.. First of all, the aerobic walking at 3.5 mph in the Fit-Step® plan burns approximately 350 calories per hour or 235 calories every 35 minutes. The strength training exercises in the Diet Fit-Step plan burn an additional 200 calories per hour or approximately 100 extra calories every 30 minutes, which is accomplished just by increasing the body's basal metabolism. So you see you can actually lose more weight, more quickly by walking with hand-held weights.

4. WHO BENEFITS FROM WALKING WITH WEIGHTS?

Studies reported at the 2008 Experimental Biology Meeting, showed that short, simple, weight-training workouts helped *men and women of all ages* lose weight and keep that weight off permanently. Weight-training also was shown to strengthen the body's immune system, as well as lower the blood pressure. By following a low-fat, moderate protein and complex carbohydrate diet, combined with simple weight-training exercises for fourteen weeks, the participants in this study lost fat and weight, and increased the proportion of muscle to body weight. Also, these men and women showed significant improvements in blood pressure, heart rate, and aerobic fitness.

Another similar study showed that middle-aged and elderly people developed stronger muscles and a healthier immune system while walking regularly, combined with light weight-training exercises. Many of the middle-aged and elderly people in this study were moderately obese when they started the program. After twelve weeks, the majority of the obese participants had lost considerable weight, in addition to gaining lean muscle mass. These individuals also developed improved cardiovascular fitness, in addition to gaining muscle strength and boosting their energy levels.

5. WHO SHOULD NOT WALK WITH WEIGHTS?

Individuals with has a medical condition such as coronary artery disease, heart disease, severe hypertension, cerebral or vascular disease and any other medical condition that their physician feels would be contraindicated by walking with weights. Also, people who have a neurological disorder, a degenerative or neuromuscular disease, or severe arthritis in any joint or in the spine should not walk with weights. In general, anyone who participates in the Diet Fit-Step Plan, with or without walking with weight, should first have a complete medical examination from their physician.

6. Improve Strength and Muscle Tone

The Fit-Step strength-training plan is a walking aerobic exercise combined with an upper body strength-training exercise. As you walk with hand-held weights, you will burn an additional 25% more calories than you would by just walking. Walking with hand-held weights also builds lean muscle mass, which burns an additional 50 calories per hour for every one pound of muscle. Walking with weights also helps develop good muscle tone, which helps improve balance and stability as you walk. Lastly, walking with weights helps develop strong arm, shoulder, chest and abdominal wall muscles, which significantly improves your posture.

7. Boost Energy and Improve Fitness

Fit-Step strength-training is the ideal combination of an aerobic walking exercise combined with strength training using hand-held weights. It is not necessary to go to the gym in order to lift heavy weights (free weights or machine operated weights) or to engage in strenuous aerobic exercises. Just by simply walking with hand-held weights 3 days per week for 35 minutes, you can achieve maximum cardiovascular fitness, burn calories, lose weight, and improve your lean body muscle mass. You will increase your metabolic rate as you burn fat, lose weight and boost your energy level. This combination of the aerobic fat-burning exercise of walking and the strength-training exercise of hand-held weights is what causes you to lose weight quickly, develop a lean firm figure and develop strong bones and muscles. This plan will also help to improve cardiovascular fitness, lower blood pressure and reduce the incidence of heart disease and strokes.

THE FIT-STEP WALKING WORKOUT

1. NATURAL ARM SWING

This is the most common arm motion that you will use naturally when walking. When you just walk without weights your arms fall into a natural, not forced, swing at the side of your body. When you walk with hand-held-weights, your arms should also hang down at your side close to your body, holding the weights with your palms facing your body. As you walk, alternately swing your arms gently, as you bend your elbows ever so slightly. This is the natural arm swing motion of walking that you will be using all of the time during your regular 6 day per week, 35 minute Fit-Step walking plan. This is a natural arm swing that is a motion that is most comfortable for you. Using the hand-held weights with this simple arm swing motion strengthens your triceps and upper shoulder muscles.

2. LOCOMOTIVE ARM MOTION

This is the arm motion that you see runners or fast walkers use. Hold your arms close to your body and bend your arms at approximately a 90 degree angle at the elbow, so your hands are making a slight fist facing in front of you. Hold the weights with palms facing your body. Now, do the locomotive! Start to move your arms alternately forward and backward. This motion strengthens the muscles of your upper arm, triceps and shoulder muscles.

Just do this exercise for a few minutes at a time during your 35 minute walk, and then go back to the natural arm swing. You can increase the number of minutes that you do the Locomotive Arm Motion as you develop more upper body strength, after you've been walking with weights for many weeks. Do not continue with this exercise if it initially causes muscle strain or pain. If you just work into it very gently, you will be able to build upper body strength gradually.

3. Hammer Curl Swing

This exercise begins exactly like the first natural arm swing exercise. Keep your arms hanging down at your sides close to your body, holding the weights with your palms facing your body. As you walk, bend each arm alternately at the elbow, towards your shoulder, and then lower each arm to the side of your body. Be sure to keep your arms close to your body. Pretend you're hammering a nail into a piece of wood or banging your fists on to a table top. This exercise strengthens your forearm and biceps muscles.

It is important to only do this exercise for a few minutes at a time during your 35 minute walk. Gradually build up the number of minutes using the Hammer Curl as you slowly improve your upper body strength over a period of many weeks on the Diet Fit-Step Plan. Remember to revert to the Natural Arm Swing motion when you stop the Hammer Curl. Discontinue this exercise if it causes any pain or strain on your muscles and try it again at a later date.

This exercise is much safer to do while walking than is the traditional biceps curl, where your palms face away from your body and your wrists are rotated outward. You will prevent the hand-held weights from bumping your legs as you walk when you do the hammer curl instead of the traditional biceps curl. Also, you get better muscle strengthening and toning with this exercise.

More Advanced Walking Workouts

The previous three exercises are the basic walking with weights exercises. Once you've become comfortable with these, say after 6-8 weeks, you can begin to try the more advanced walking with hand-held weights exercises (#4, 5 and 6). If these appear too difficult or strenuous to do while you're walking, do them at the end of your 35 minute walk, when you are standing still. Remember to gradually build up these exercises slowly, until you reach a point where you're comfortable doing them without any strain on your body.

4. REACH FOR THE SKY

Bend your arms at the side of your body with your elbows bent and pointing towards your feet. Hold the weights in your hands, palms facing your body at shoulder level. Do not turn your wrists outwards as weight-lifters do when they lift heavy weights. Raise the weights above head, until arms are fully extended. Then lower weights back down to shoulder level. Again, do this exercise for only a few minutes at a time during your 35 minute walking workout. This exercise can slowly be increased as you continue to build upper body strength over a period of many weeks on the Diet Fit-Step plan. Again remember to discontinue the Reach for the Sky exercise if it causes pain or strain in your muscles.

Now, reach for the sky! Think of this exercise as lifting the weight of the world off of your shoulders as you reach for the sky. This exercise sculpts and strengthens the upper back and shoulder muscles.

5. FLAP YOUR WINGS

Hold the weights next to the sides of your legs, palms facing in. Lift both arms together, out to your sides and away from your body. Lift arms out away from your body, to just slightly below the level of your shoulders (never any higher) as you walk, then lower both arms to your sides. This exercise must be done carefully while you're walking; otherwise you may lose your balance or knock into someone or something that is next to you. Remember to only do this exercise for a few minutes at a time and then revert to the Natural Arm Swing motion for the rest of your 35 minute Fit-Step walk. As with exercise #4, if you find that this exercise is too difficult to do while walking, wait until your walk is finished and then do 10-12 repetitions of the Flap Your Wings exercise. This exercise strengthens your upper back, chest and shoulder muscles.

6. BUTTERFLY STROKE

Hold weights in each hand in front of you at chest level, palms facing each other and your elbows bent at 90 degrees pointing towards your feet. Spread both arms out to your sides like a butterfly, being careful not to spread your arms out too wide past your shoulder level. Then bring the weights back together in front of you at chest level. Be careful not to bang your hands or the weights together. You can also vary this exercise by extending your arms directly in front of you, then spread your arms out to your sides and then bring them back together. Only do this exercise for a few minutes if you try it while walking and then revert to the Natural Arm Swing motion for the rest of your 35 minute walk. As with any of the other exercises, stop this one also if you feel pain or strain in your muscles. As you gradually build your upper body strength you can try this exercise slowly and gently during or after your 35 minute walk. This exercise is particularly good for strengthening, developing and sculpting mid-chest and upper back muscles.

If you find this exercise is too difficult to do while walking, then you can do it at the end of your 35-minute walk. If you're tired, you can even do this exercise lying down as follows:

a. Lie on your back, with your knees bent and your feet flat on the floor.

b. Start with arms stretched out above you towards the ceiling with weights in each hand, with palms facing each other.

c. Slowly lower your arms out to the sides, and then gently pull arms back to starting positions directly above and in front of you. Use primarily your chest muscles while doing this exercise, not your arm muscles.

FIT-STEP WORKOUT EXERCISE TIPS

1. **Start with 1-pound weights** in each hand three times per week for the first 21 days, and then you can build up to 2-pound weights after you feel comfortable walking with 1-pound weights. If you find however, that 2-pound weights are too heavy, then stick with the 1-pound weights. Studies show that you still will get the same great muscle strengthening, toning and sculpting with very light weights. Actually most people do just fine with one pound weights.

2. **The first three main Fit-Step Exercises** only have to be done 2 days per week when you first start walking with weights to achieve maximum strength training and muscle toning benefits. If the weather is bad, these exercises can be done at home. Only do one set of 10-12 repetitions of each exercise, after your 35-minute workout indoors while standing still. After you've been doing these exercises for 14 days or more, you can build up to two to three sets of 10-12 repetitions per week, while walking or while standing still after your 35 minute walk. After 21 days you can start to walk three times per week using hand-held weights for increased calorie burning and improved muscle tone.

3. **Only try exercises # 4, 5 and 6** when you've become thoroughly conditioned, after you've completed 21 or more days on the Fit-Step strength-training exercise plan. You can vary the exercises as you walk. Remember to stop any particular exercise if you become tired or your muscles become sore or feel strained. Remember, these exercises can be done at the end of your 35 minute walk, if you find them too difficult to do while walking. Start with one set of 10-12 repetitions of each exercise at the end of your walk and then you can build them up to two or three sets of 10-12 repetitions after you've completed the first 21 or more days on your Fit-Step Exercise walking plan.

4. **Tighten your abdominal muscles** intermittently while you're doing these exercises, whether you're walking or standing still. This helps to provide support for your upper body and back, while helping to trim, tone and flatten your abdominal muscles.

5. **How would you like to lighten your load** as you continue on your Fit-Step 35 minute walk? Instead of using hand-held weights, you can occasionally carry one 24 ounce plastic bottle of water in each hand. As you proceed on your 35-minute walk, you can drink from each bottle alternately, until each bottles becomes lighter and lighter. When you're finished with your workout, you will be refreshed and rehydrated.

6. How Many Repetitions Should You Do With Each Exercise?
You'll be able to customize the number of repetitions for each exercise depending on your own comfort level. During the first 21 days on the Diet Fit-Step Plan, it's only necessary to do one set of 10-12 repetitions for each exercise. This is usually adequate strength training, as you rotate from one exercise to another. Then you should revert to your Natural Arm Swing motion of walking for the rest of your walk. Remember to start slowly with fewer repetitions when you start your walking workout and gradually build up the number of repetitions until you reach your comfort level. You can gradually increase the number of repetitions after the first 3 weeks depending on your level of comfort.

7. How Often Should You Walk With Weights?
Many studies in exercise physiology show that strength training exercises two or three days per week, will prevent damage to muscle fibers that need time to heal after being stressed with weight resistance exercises. Also, by varying the strength-training exercises to different muscle groups, it helps to provide exercise to all of the upper body's muscles on a graduated basis. The significance of the Fit-Step Strength Training exercises (# 1, 2 and 3) is that they are done while you are walking using very light weights. This considerably decreases the likelihood of muscle and ligament injury and eliminates the need to go to the gym for time-consuming, back-breaking, weight lifting routines. The latest research in exercise physiology has definitely shown that working-out different muscle groups only two or three times a week offers the same strength and muscle-firming benefits, as working out these muscle groups three or four times per week.

Therefore, on your regular Fit-Step plan, you will be walking for 35 minutes, six days per week. In the beginning, it will only be necessary to use hand-held weights on two days each week on your walking workout. As you continue your Fit-Step walking with weights program, you can increase the number of days to three days per week after the first 21 days. Your walking workout with hand-held weights, three times per week will then result in more muscle toning, sculpting and strengthening. We've found that walking with lightweight (1-2 lbs.), hand-held weights three times per week is preferable over the long run to twice weekly, since it definitely helps weight-loss and weight-maintenance, in addition to upper body strength-training.

8. Make up Your Own Individual Strength-Training Exercises
Remember, if you find that walking with hand-held weights three times per week is too difficult, or if you feel that it causes you too much exertion, then decrease walking with weights to two times per week. If you feel that walking with weight is altogether too uncomfortable, do the workout exercises with the weights after your 35 minute walk, while you are standing at rest. On average, you should alternate each exercise one time (one set) with 10 to12 repetitions each. You can devise your own number of repetitions for each of the exercises depending on how you feel, and you can also increase the number of sets that you do the exercises over a period of time, depending on how you feel. Don't push yourself. Don't tire your muscles or yourself, just set your own individual pace so you're comfortable with the strength-training exercises. Stop if you have a backache or if you develop any other pain or discomfort anywhere in your body or if you develop any other symptoms. Check with your doctor if you have any questions or concerns.

9. The Easy Body-Shaping Workout
This workout does not involve lifting heavy free weights or working with complicated weight-machines at the gym. This easy plan features a unique combination of 35-minutes of aerobic exercise—walking six days per week, combined with walking three days per week, using light, hand-held weights for strength-training. These light weights strengthen and build upper body muscles and bones as you walk, while burning additional calories by boosting your body's metabolism. This combination of an aerobic exercise and strength training delivers a double-blast of calorie burning, for complete cardiovascular fitness, maximum weight-loss and complete body-shaping.

10. Make sure that you get a **complete physical examination** from your own physician before starting any phase of the Diet Fit-Step Plan, including the strength-training exercises.

What's the Best Time To Do the Fit-Step Workout?

You can do your walking aerobic workout exercise any time of the day that's convenient for you. It's your schedule, so make it any time that you'd like. You can also change the times that you exercise each day depending on your own individual work schedule or home activities. Here are the pros and cons of exercising at various times of the day according to the so-called fitness experts. Take it with a grain of salt and individualize your schedule to your own liking.

Morning – The main obstacle in the morning is getting out of bed. Once you're up, depending on if you're an early riser or not, you may want to leave yourself enough time so that you won't be rushed, especially if you have to go to work or have home responsibilities. Since there are usually few disruptions in the A.M., women and men who walk in the morning are more likely to stick with their exercise plans over a long period of time. Plus, the sense of accomplishment, having completed your exercise early in the day, gives you a psychological rush for the first part of the day.

Afternoon – Many people feel an energy lag between two and three P.M. in the afternoon, which is related to the body's natural circadian rhythm. It may also be partly due to having just eaten lunch. Some exercise physiologists say that walking mid-day can smooth out that energy lag by increasing the levels of certain hormones that will perk you up for several hours. Remember, however, that it is not a good idea to exercise immediately after lunch or to skip lunch altogether. Walking for 35 minutes and then eating a light lunch will boost your energy level for the rest of the day.

Evening – Due to fluctuations in biological rhythms, it is in the late afternoon or early evening when your breathing is easier because your lungs' airways open wider, your muscle strength increases due to a slightly higher body temperature, and your joints and muscles are at their most flexible. This may also be a good time to walk according to some exercise physiologists. However, if you've had an extremely difficult day, and if you're dead tired, then revving yourself up for exercise may seem more like a chore than fun. Also, never exercise near bedtime, since the increased energy levels that follow the exercise may make it difficult to fall asleep. Determine the best time to do your workout according to your own biological clock and how you feel, and also according to your own time schedule. It's your body, so listen to it, and it will respond to you with boundless energy and pep when you do the Diet Fit-Step Plan.

Once You're Fit, It Takes Longer to Get Out of Shape

What if I can't keep up with the exercise plan regularly? What if I have to stop for a few days or a week or even longer if some interruption in my life prevents me from continuing? This is the kind of thinking that prevents many men and women from starting an exercise program and prevents others from going back to one that they've already begun. Never fear, the answer's here—**"It takes much longer to get out of shape than it does to get into shape."**

The Diet Fit-Step Plan is forgiving. Even if you miss a few days or a week or a few weeks in a month, there is no need to worry. Once you have been conditioned physically, it takes a lot longer to get out of shape than it took you to get into shape. The rate of regression depends on how long you've been exercising and how fit you are. The body is remarkable, since it tends to hold on to these fitness gains long after you've stopped exercising. Most women and men lose muscle strength at about one-half the rate at which they gained it. So, if you've been doing your aerobic walking program and your strength-training exercises for three months, and have to discontinue for any reason, it could take up to six months for your body to fall back to its pre-training state.

Aerobic capacity starts to decrease in the first two to three weeks after you've stopped exercising, but it can take almost six to eight months before fit exercisers get back to the fitness level where they started. Aerobic exercising (walking) decreases the LDL (bad cholesterol) and increases the HDL (good cholesterol) after you've been on your walking program for approximately two to three months. Studies show that it took at least three months for these cholesterol levels to return to their original pre-walking workout levels after the exercise of walking was discontinued.

That's pretty good, considering you've stopped walking all that time. When walkers resume their walking program, it took them only one-half the time to return to their original levels of fitness. So, don't worry if you have to discontinue your walking program for any reason or for any period of time. The benefits that you've worked so hard for are long-lasting and are easily obtained again in half the time. **The Diet Fit-Step Plan is forgiving and it keeps on giving!**

CARDIO AND STRENGTH TRAINING COMBO

When you combine a cardiovascular workout with strength training exercises into one exercise routine, you save time, which is a great factor for most people whose time is limited.

Secondly, this cardio and strength training combo boosts the cardiovascular benefits and increases the aerobic calorie burning from walking, while doing upper body exercises. This double-blast of calorie-burning increases the amount of weight that you can lose in one half the time, not to mention the added health benefits of improved cardiovascular fitness.

Walking with light-weight, hand-held weights is the perfect effective combination for cardiovascular and strength training. Unfortunately, there are some people who have tried to vary this cardio strength training exercise using elastic arm bands wrapped around the console of a treadmill or an elliptical machine. This strenuous combination can increase your heartbeat and breathing too rapidly and puts excessive stress on your cardiovascular system. These elastic bands could also affect your normal gait on a treadmill, and will cause you to burn fewer calories because this activity will make you slow down. In addition, this awkward exercise combination can cause added stress and strain in your upper body's ligaments and tendons, and make you more prone to stress injuries.

Also, elliptical machines, stationary bikes, treadmills with arm levers that pull back and push forward, do very little to develop upper body strength. They only provide passive motion for your upper arms and can actually interfere with your normal gait and cause shoulder and upper body and arm injuries.

There's no doubt that the safest, easiest and most effective cardio-strength combination is the strength-training component of the Fit-Step plan. Walking for 35 minutes, 3 days per week with light-weight, hand-held weights develops maximum cardiovascular fitness and upper body strength training. This power combo burns additional calories for weight loss, tones your muscles, and shapes your figure.

THE FINAL CLUE

You'll be able to stay motivated when you add the Diet Fit-Step Strength-Training Exercises to your 35 minute walk, since you'll be walking for 35 minutes with light-weight, hand-held weight three times per week. These strength-training exercises help to build your upper body muscles as you burn extra calories. By using different upper body muscles while walking with hand-held weights, you'll be able to stay motivated by varying your exercise routine. You will feel stronger and have more energy as your metabolic rate increases with this additional muscle activity. You in fact, have a double burst of calorie burning with the Diet Fit-Step walking with weights plan. First you'll burn calories by the aerobic activity of walking and secondly you'll burn additional calories by building additional muscle tissue which actively burns calories. This double blast of calorie burning promotes maximum weight-loss, physical fitness and body shaping.

This third component of the Diet Fit-Step Plan is the *final and vital clue* in this mystery weight-loss and fitness plan, which helps you to lose weight, stay fit, and build strong bones and muscles.

You will boost your energy level, as your metabolic rate increases, and you will burn more calories as you walk with hand-held weights. You will also develop maximum cardiovascular fitness and develop a shapely, more sculptured body. The three combined clues are the keys to the *Diet Fit-Step Mystery Plan* set forth herein, in *The Case of the Unwanted Pounds*. You will slim-down, shape-up, look younger, and live longer on this unique weight-loss and fitness plan. And you will finally *shed those unwanted pounds permanently,* that have been plaguing you all of these years.

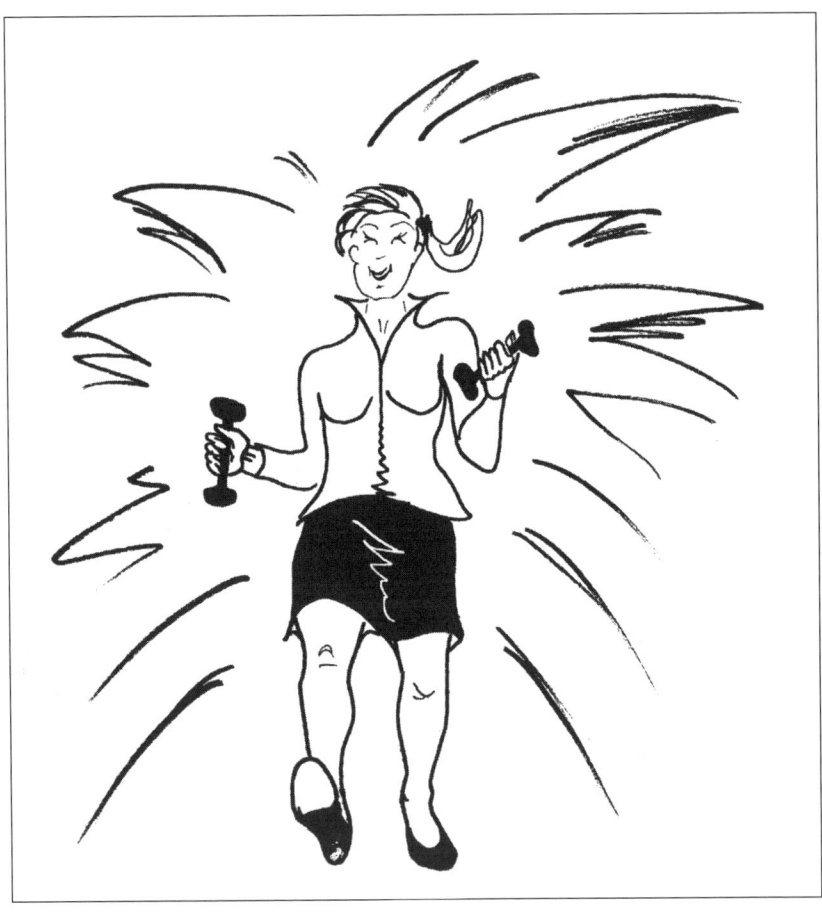

Appendix
Fat & Fiber Counter

Sources of Information

- United States Department of Agriculture
- Center for Science and Public Interest
- Food Manufacturers, Processors and Distributors
- Bowes and Church's Food Values of Portions Commonly Used (Pennington and Church, 17th Ed.)
- Scientific Journals and Publications
- Author Extrapolations

Interpreting Food Labels

- Sugar Free: Less than ½ gram sugar per serving
- Calorie Free: No more than 5 calories per serving
- Salt Free: Less than 5 milligrams of sodium per serving
- Low Sodium: No more than 140 milligrams of sodium per serving
- Fat Free: Less than ½ gram fat per serving
- Low-fat: No more than 3 grams fat per serving
- Reduced fat: At least 25% less fat than comparison food
- Low Saturated Fat: No more than 1 gram saturated fat per serving
- Reduced Saturated Fat: No more than 50% saturated fat of comparison food
- Light: ½ the fat in or ⅓ fewer calories than the regular version of a similar food

BREAD AND FLOUR

Item	Serving	Tot. Fat (g)	Sat. Fat (g)	Chol. (mg)	Fiber (g)
Bagel, Plain	1 medium	1.1	0.2	0	2
Bagel, Cinnamon Raisin	1 medium	1.2	0.2	0	2
Barley Flour	1 cup	0.5	1.3	0	3
Biscuit					
Plain	1 medium	6.6	1.9	3	1
Buttermilk	1 medium	5.8	0.9	2	1
From Mix	1 medium	4.3	1.2	3	1
Bread					
Cracked Wheat	1 slice	1.0	0.2	0	1
French/Vienna	1 slice	1.0	0.2	0	1
Italian	1 slice	0.5	0.1	0	1
Matzoh	1 piece	0.5	0.1	0	0
Mixed Grain	1 slice	0.9	0.2	0	2
Multigrain, "Lite"	1 slice	0.5	0.0	2	3
Pita, Plain	1 large	0.7	0.1	0	2
Pita, Whole Wheat	1 large	1.2	0.3	0	4
Pumpernickel	1 slice	0.8	0.0	0	2
Raisin	1 slice	1.1	0.3	0	1
Rye	1 slice	0.9	0.2	0	2
Sourdough	1 slice	0.8	0.2	0	1
Wheat, Commercial	1 slice	1.1	0.3	0	2
Wheat, "Lite"	1 slice	0.5	0.1	0	3
White, Commercial	1 slice	1.0	0.2	0	0
White, "Lite"	1 slice	0.5	0.1	0	1
Whole Wheat, Commercial	1 slice	1.2	0.3	0	3
Bread Crumbs	1 cup	1.5	1.3	0	2
Breadsticks	2 small	0.5	0.2	0	0
Bulgar	½ cup	2.0	0.3	0	5.2
Cornbread	1 piece	5.5	2.0	12	1.5
Cornmeal, Dry	½ cup	2.3	0.3	0	6
Cornstarch	1 T	0.0	0.0	0	0
Crackers					
Cheese	5 pieces	4.9	1.6	4	0
Cheese Nips	13 crackers	3.2	1.2	3	0
Cheese w/Peanut Bttr	2 oz. Pkg.	13.5	2.9	7	1
Goldfish, Any Flavor	12 crackers	2.0	0.7	1	0

Item	Serving	Tot. Fat (g)	Sat. Fat (g)	Chol. (mg)	Fiber (g)
Crackers (continued)					
Graham	2 squares	1.3	0.4	0	0
Harvest Wheats	4 crackers	3.6	1.1	0	1
Melba Toast	1 piece	0.2	0.0	0	0
Oyster	15 crackers	2.1	0.3	0	0
Rice Cakes	1 piece	0.2	0.2	0	0
Ritz	3 crackers	3.0	3.0	1	0
Ritz Cheese	3 crackers	3.9	3.9	2	0
Ryekrisp, Plain	2 crackers	0.2	0.2	0	2
Ryekrisp, Sesame	2 crackers	1.4	1.4	0	3
Saltines	2 crackers	0.7	0.7	0	0
Sesame Wafers	3 crackers	3.0	3.0	0	0
Snackwell's Wheat	5 crackers	0.0	0.0	0	1
Sociables	6 crackers	3.0	3.0	0	0
Soda	5 crackers	1.9	1.9	0	0
Tsted w/Peanut Butter	1.5 oz. Pkg.	10.5	10.5	2	0
Triscuit	2 crackers	1.6	1.6	0	1
Vegetable Thins	7 crackers	4.0	4.0	0	0
Wheat Thins	4 crackers	1.5	1.5	0	0
Wheat w/Cheese	1.5 oz. Pkg.	10.9	10.9	1	0
Crepe	1 medium	12.5	12.5	37	0
Croissant	1 medium	11.5	11.5	30	1
Croutons, Commercial	¼ cup	1.8	1.8	0	1
Danish Pastry	1 medium	19.3	19.3	30	1
Doughnut					
Cake	(1) 2 oz.	16.2	16.2	24	1
Yeast	(1) 2 oz.	13.3	13.3	21	1
English Muffin					
Plain	1	1.1	1.1	0	1
w/Raisins	1	1.2	1.2	0	1
Whole Wheat	1	2.0	2.0	0	2
Flour					
Buckwheat	1 cup	3.0	3.0	0	8
Rice	1 cup	1.3	1.3	0	3
Rye	1 cup	2.2	2.2	0	11
Soy	1 cup	16.0	16.0	0	4
White, All Purpose	1 cup	1.2	1.2	0	4
Whole Wheat	1 cup	2.3	2.3	0	12

BREAD AND FLOUR (CONTINUED)

Item	Serving	Tot. Fat (g)	Sat. Fat (g)	Chol. (mg)	Fiber (g)
French Toast					
Frzn Variety	1 slice	6.0	6.0	54	0
Hmde	1 slice	10.7	10.7	75	1
Funnel Cake	4 in. diam.	12.8	12.8	48	1
Muffins					
Banana Nut	1 medium	5.0	2.2	20	2
Blueberry, From Mix	1 medium	5.1	1.1	9	1
Bran, Hmde	1 medium	5.8	1.2	16	3
Corn	1 medium	4.8	0.9	18	2
White, Plain	1 medium	5.4	1.1	12	1
Pancakes					
Blueberry, From Mix	3 medium	15.0	4.3	80	4
Buckwheat, From Mix	3 medium	12.3	3.9	75	3
Buttermilk, From Mix	3 medium	10.0	3.2	80	2
"Lite," From Mix	3 medium	2.0	0.6	20	5
Whole Wht, From Mix	3 medium	3.0	1.0	30	6
Phyllo Dough	2 oz.	6.4	0.5	0	1
Pie Crust, Plain	1/8 pie	8.0	1.9	0	0
Popover	1	5.0	2.6	51	0
Rolls					
Crescent	1	5.6	2.8	6	1
Croissant	1 small	6.0	3.5	21	0
French	1	0.4	0.1	0	1
Hamburger	1	3.0	0.8	1	1
Hard	1	1.2	0.3	1	1
Hot Dog	1	2.1	0.5	1	1
Kaiser	1 medium	2.0	0.5	0	0
Raisin	1 large	1.9	0.5	0	1
Rye, Dark	1	1.6	0.1	0	2
Rye, Light, Hard	1	1.0	0.1	0	2
Sandwich	1	3.1	0.4	2	1
Sesame Seed	1	2.1	0.6	1	1
Sourdough	1	1.0	0.0	0	1
Submarine/Hoagie	1 medium	3.0	0.8	3	2
Wheat	1	1.7	0.4	0	1
White, Commercial	1	2.2	1.0	1	0
Whole Wheat	1	1.1	0.2	1	3

Item	Serving	Tot. Fat (g)	Sat. Fat (g)	Chol. (mg)	Fiber (g)
Scone	1	5.5	1.5	28	1
Soft Pretzel	1 medium	1.5	0.7	2	1.5
Stuffing					
Bread, From Mix	½ cup	12.2	6.0	0	0
Cornbread, From Mix	½ cup	4.8	2.5	43	0
Stove Top	½ cup	9.0	5.0	21	0
Sweet Roll, Iced	1 medium	7.9	2.1	20	1
Toaster Pastry	1	5.0	0.8	0	0
Tortilla					
Corn (Unfried)	1 medium	1.1	0.2	0	1
Flour	1 medium	2.5	1.1	0	1
Turnover, Fruit Filled	1	15.0	3.7	0	1
Waffle					
Frozen	1 medium	3.2	0.8	11	1
Hmde	1 medium	9.5	4.1	50	1
From Mix	1 medium	8.5	3.0	48	1

CEREALS

Item	Serving	Tot. Fat (g)	Sat. Fat (g)	Chol. (mg)	Fiber (g)
All Bran	⅓ cup	0.5	0.1	0	10
Apple Jacks	1 cup	0.1	0.0	0	1
Bran, 100%	½ cup	1.9	0.3	0	9
Bran Chex	1 cup	1.2	0.2	0	9
Bran Flakes, 40%	1 cup	0.7	0.1	0	6
Cheerios	1 cup	1.6	0.3	0	2
Cocoa Krispies	1 cup	0.5	0.2	0	0
Corn Chex	1 cup	0.1	0.0	0	1
Cornflakes	1 cup	0.1	0.0	0	1
Cracklin' Oat Bran	⅓ cup	2.7	1.3	0	3
Cream of Wheat w/o Fat	½ cup	0.3	0.0	0	0
Crispix	1 cup	0.0	0.0	0	1
Fiber One	1 cup	2.0	0.4	0	13
Frosted Bran, Kellogg's	¾ cup	0.0	0.0	0	3
Frosted Mini-Wheats	4 biscuits	0.3	0.0	0	1
Fruit and Fiber w/Dates, Raisins					
Walnuts	⅔ cup	2.0	0.3	0	5
w/Peaches, Almonds	⅔ cup	2.0	0.3	0	5

Cereals (continued)

Item	Serving	Tot. Fat (g)	Sat. Fat (g)	Chol. (mg)	Fiber (g)
Fruitful Bran	⅔ cup	0.0	0.0	0	5
Fruit Loops	1 cup	0.5	0.0	0	1
Golden Grahams	¾ cup	1.1	0.1		1
Granola					
Commercial Brands	⅓ cup	4.9	1.8	0	3
Low-Fat, Kellogg's	⅓ cup	2.0	0.0	0	2
Grapenut Flakes	1 cup	0.4	0.2	0	2
Grapenuts	¼ cup	0.1	0.0	0	2
Life, Plain Or Cinn.	1 cup	2.5	0.5	0	4
Mueslix, Kellogg's	½ cup	1.0	0.8	0	5
Nutri-Grain, Kellogg's					
Almond Raisin	⅔ cup	2.0	0.4	0	3
Raisin Bran	1 cup	1.0	0.1	0	5
Wheat	⅔ cup	0.3	0.0	0	3
Oat Bran, Cooked Cereal					
w/o Added Fat	½ cup	0.5	0.1	0	2
Oats					
Instant	1 packet	1.7	0.2	0	1
w/o Added Fat	½ cup	1.2	0.2	0	1
Product 19	1 cup	0.2	0.0	0	1
Puffed Rice	1 cup	0.2	0.0	0	1
Puffed Wheat	1 cup	0.1	0.0	0	1
Raisin Bran	1 cup	0.8	0.1	0	5
Rice Chex	1 cup	0.1	0.0	0	1
Rice Krispies	1 cup	0.2	0.0	0	0
Shredded Wheat	1 cup	0.3	0.0	0	2
Special K	1 cup	0.1	0.0	0	0
Sugar Frosted Flakes	1 cup	0.5	0.1	0	1
Total	1 cup	0.7	0.1	0	2
Total Raisin Bran	1 cup	1.0	0.1	0	5
Wheat Chex	1 cup	1.2	0.2	0	6
Wheaties	1 cup	0.5	0.1	0	2

Dairy Products (Cheeses)

Item	Serving	Tot. Fat (g)	Sat. Fat (g)	Chol. (mg)	Fiber (g)
American					
Processed	1 oz.	8.9	5.6	27	0
Reduced Calorie	1 oz.	2.0	1.0	12	0
Blue	1 oz.	8.2	5.3	21	0
Borden's Fat Free	1 oz.	<0.5	<0.3	<5	0
Borden's Lite Line	1 oz.	2.0	<1.0	NA	0
Caraway	1 oz.	8.3	5.4	30	0
Cheddar	1 oz.	9.2	5.0	26	0
Cheese Sauce	¼ cup	9.8	4.3	20	0
Cheese Spread, Kraft	1 oz.	6.0	3.8	16	0
Cheez Whiz	1 oz.	6.0	3.1	16	0
Cottage Cheese					
1% Fat	½ cup	1.2	0.8	5	0
2% Fat	½ cup	2.2	1.4	10	0
Creamed	½ cup	5.1	3.2	17	0
Cream Cheese					
Kraft Free	1 oz. (2T)	0.0	0.0	5	0
Lite	1 oz. (2T)	6.6	4.2	20	0
Regular	1 oz. (2T)	9.9	6.2	31	0
Edam	1 oz.	7.9	5.0	25	0
Feta	1 oz.	6.0	4.2	25	0
Gouda	1 oz.	7.8	5.0	32	0
Jarlsberg	1 oz.	6.9	4.2	16	0
Kraft American Singles	1 oz.	7.5	4.3	25	0
Kraft Free Singles	1 oz.	0.0	0.0	5	0
Kraft Light Singles	1 oz.	4.0	2.0	15	0
Light N'lively Singles	1 oz.	4.0	2.0	15	0
Monterey Jack	1 oz.	8.6	5.0	30	0
Mozzarella					
Part Skim	1 oz.	4.5	2.4	16	0
Whole Milk	1 oz.	6.1	3.7	22	0
Muenster	1 oz.	8.5	5.4	27	0
Parmesan					
Grated	1 T	1.5	1.0	4	0
Hard	1 oz.	7.3	4.7	19	0
Pimento Cheese Spread	1 oz.	8.9	5.6	27	0

Dairy Products (Cheeses) continued

Item	Serving	Tot. Fat (g)	Sat. Fat (g)	Chol. (mg)	Fiber (g)
Provolone	1 oz.	7.6	4.8	20	0
Ricotta					
"Lite" Reduced Fat	½ cup	4.0	2.4	15	0
Part Skim	½ cup	9.8	6.1	38	0
Whole Milk	½ cup	16.1	10.3	63	0
Romano	1 oz.	7.6	4.9	29	0
Roquefort	1 oz.	7.8	5.0	24	0
Swiss					
Alpine Lace	1 oz.	1.5	0.5	5	0
Sliced	1 oz.	7.8	5.0	26	0
Velveeta	1 oz.	7.0	4.0	20	0
Velveeta Light	1 oz.	4.0	2.0	15	0

Eggs

Item	Serving	Tot. Fat (g)	Sat. Fat (g)	Chol. (mg)	Fiber (g)
Boiled-Poached	1	5.6	1.6	213	0
Fried w/ ½ T Margarine	1 large	7.6	2.7	240	0
Omelet					
2 Oz. Cheese, 3 Egg	1	37.0	12.3	480	0
Plain, 3 Egg	1	21.3	5.2	430	0
Spanish, 2 Egg	1	18.0	5.9	375	1
Scrambled w/Milk	1 large	8.0	2.8	214	0
Substitute, Frzn	¼ cup	0.0	0.0	0	0
White	1 large	0.0	0.0	0	0
Yolk	1 large	5.6	1.6	213	0

MILK AND YOGURT

Item	Serving	Tot. Fat (g)	Sat. Fat (g)	Chol. (mg)	Fiber (g)
Buttermilk					
1% Fat	1 cup	2.2	1.3	9	0
Dry	1 T	0.4	0.2	5	0
Chocolate Milk					
2% Fat	1 cup	5.0	3.1	17	0
Whole	1 cup	8.5	5.3	30	0
Evaporated Milk					
Skim	½ cup	0.4	0.0	0	0
Whole	½ cup	9.5	5.8	37	0
Hot Cocoa					
Mix w/Water	1 cup	3.0	0.7	5	0
w/Skim Milk	1 cup	2.0	0.9	12	0
w/Whole Milk	1 cup	9.1	5.6	33	0
Low-fat Milk					
½% Fat	1 cup	1.0	4.0	10	0
1% Fat	1 cup	2.6	1.6	10	0
2% Fat	1 cup	4.7	2.9	18	0
Milkshake					
Choc. Thick	1 cup	6.1	3.8	24	1
Vanilla, Thick	1 cup	6.9	4.3	27	0
Skim Milk					
Liquid	1 cup	0.4	0.3	4	0
Nonfat Dry Powder	¼ cup	0.2	0.2	6	0
Whole Milk					
3.5% Fat	1 cup	8.2	5.0	34	0
Dry Powder	¼ cup	8.6	5.4	31	0
Yogurt					
Frzn, Low-fat	½ cup	3.0	2.0	10	0
Frzn, Nonfat	½ cup	0.2	0.0	0	0
Fruit Flavored, Low-fat	1 cup	2.6	0.1	10	0
Plain Yogurt					
Low-fat	1 cup	3.5	2.3	14	0
Skim (Nonfat)	1 cup	0.4	0.3	4	0
Whole Milk	1 cup	7.4	4.8	29	0

Desserts

Item	Serving	Tot. Fat (g)	Sat. Fat (g)	Chol. (mg)	Fiber (g)
Apple Betty	½ cup	13.3	2.7	0	3
Baklava	1 piece	29.2	7.2	7	2
Brownie					
Choc., Plain	1	5.0	1.5	14	0
Choc. w/Frosting	1	9.0	1.5	20	1
Choc. w/Nuts	1	7.3	1.8	10	1
Cake					
Angel Food	1/8 cake	0.1	0.0	0	0
Banana	1/8 cake	14.5	2.5	50	1
Black Forest	1/8 cake	15.0	2.0	50	1
Carrot w/Frosting	1/8 cake	18.0	3.6	53	3
Choc. w/Frosting	1/8 cake	16.0	4.0	77	2
Coconut w/Frosting	1/8 cake	17.0	5.4	51	2
Coffee Cake	1/8 cake	6.1	1.0	42	1
Devil's Food, "Light" From Mix	1/8 cake	2.8	1.1	42	0
German Choc. w/ Frosting	1/8 cake	17.0	4.1	72	2
Gingerbread	1/8 cake	2.6	0.9	1.3	0
Lemon Chiffon	1/8 cake	3.0	0.7	3	0
Marble w/Frosting	1/8 cake	15.0	2.5	62	1
Pound	1/8 cake	8.2	4.0	50	1
Spice w/Frosting	1/8 cake	10.2	2.8	48	1
Sponge	1/8 cake	2.0	0.5	50	0
White w/Frosting	1/8 cake	13.1	3.0	30	1
White, "Light", From Mix	1/8 cake	2.6	0.5	15	0
Yellow, "Light", From Mix	1/8 cake	3.0	1.2	35	0
Yellow w/Frosting	1/8 cake	14.0	4.0	50	1
Cheesecake, Traditional	1/8 pie	22.0	10.4	36	0
Cobbler					
w/Biscuit Topping	½ cup	6.0	1.7	2	3
w/Pie-Crust Topping	½ cup	9.3	3.6	5	3
Cookies					
Animal	15 cookies	4.7	1.2	0	0

Fat & Fiber Counter

Item	Serving	Tot. Fat (g)	Sat. Fat (g)	Chol. (mg)	Fiber (g)
Cookies (continued)					
Chantilly, Pepperidge Farm	1	2.0	1.0	<5	0
Choc.	1	3.3	1.0	6	0
Choc. Chip Hmde	1	3.7	2.0	8	0
Choc. Chip, Pepperidge Farm	1	2.5	1.4	<5	0
Choc. Sandwich (Oreo Type)	1	2.1	0.4	0	0
Entenmann's Fat-Free	2	0.0	0.0	0	0
Fat-Free Newtons	1	0.0	0.0	0	0
Fig Bar	1	1.0	0.2	0	1
Fig Newtons	1	1.0	0.3	0	0
Gingersnap	1	1.6	0.3	0	0
Graham Cracker, Choc. Covered	1	3.1	0.9	0	0
Macaroon, Coconut	1	3.4	1.3	0	0
Oatmeal	1	3.2	0.6	0	0
Oatmeal Raisin	1	3.0	0.8	0	0
Peanut Butter	1	3.2	1.0	6	1
Rice Krispie Bar	1	0.9	0.3	0	0
Shortbread	1	2.3	0.4	2	0
Cupcake					
Choc. w/Icing	1	5.5	2.1	22	1
Yellow w/Icing	1	6.0	2.3	23	1
Custard, Baked	½ cup	6.9	3.4	123	0
Date Bar	1 bar	2.0	0.7	2	1
Dumpling, Fruit	1 piece	15.1	5.5	8	2
Éclair (With Choc. Icing & Custard)	1 small	15.4	5.7	115	0
Fruitcake	1 piece	6.2	1.4	11	1
Fruit Ice, Italian	½ cup	0.0	0.0	0	0
Fudgesicle	1 bar	0.4	0.2	3	1
Granola Bar	1 bar	6.8	1.5	0	1
Ice Cream					
Choc. (10% Fat)	½ cup	7.3	4.5	23	1
Choc. (16% Fat)	½ cup	17.0	8.9	44	0
Dietetic, Sugar-Free	½ cup	3.5	1.3	27	0
Vanilla Soft Serve	½ cup	11.3	6.4	76	0

Desserts (continued)

Item	Serving	Tot. Fat (g)	Sat. Fat (g)	Chol. (mg)	Fiber (g)
Ice Cream (continued)					
Strawberry (10% Fat)	½ cup	6.0	4.0	28	0
Vanilla (10% Fat)	½ cup	7.0	5.4	28	0
Vanilla (16% Fat)	½ cup	11.9	7.4	44	0
Ice Cream Bar					
Choc. Coated	1 bar	11.5	10.0	23	0
Toffee Crunch	1 bar	10.2	7.0	9	1
Ice Cream Cake Roll	1 slice	6.9	4.0	52	0
Ice Cream Cone (Cone Only)	1 medium	0.3	0.1	0	0
Ice Cream Drumstick	1	10.0	4.1	14	1
Ice Cream Sandwich	1	8.3	4.4	12	0
Ice Milk					
Choc.	½ cup	2.0	1.3	9	0
Soft Serve, All Flavors	½ cup	2.3	1.4	7	0
Strawberry	½ cup	2.5	1.2	7	0
Vanilla	½ cup	2.8	1.5	8	0
Jello	½ cup	0.0	0.0	0	0
Ladyfinger	1	2.0	0.5	80	0
Lemon Bars	1 bar	3.2	7.0	13	0
Mousse, Choc.	½ cup	15.5	8.7	124	1
Napoleon	1 piece	5.3	2.6	10	0
Pie					
Apple	1/8 pie	16.9	2.3	3	3
Banana Cream Or Custard	1/8 pie	14.0	10.0	35	1
Blueberry	1/8 pie	17.3	4.0	0	3
Boston Cream Pie	1/8 pie	10.0	3.1	20	1
Cherry	1/8 pie	18.1	5.0	0	2
Choc. Cream	1/8 pie	13.0	4.5	15	3
Coconut Cream Or Custard	1/8 pie	19.0	7.0	80	1
Key Lime	1/8 pie	19.0	6.8	10	1
Lemon Chiffon	1/8 pie	13.5	3.7	15	1
Lemon Meringue, Traditional	1/8 pie	13.1	5.1	50	1
Peach	1/8 pie	17.7	4.6	3	3

Item	Serving	Tot. Fat (g)	Sat. Fat (g)	Chol. (mg)	Fiber (g)
Pie (continued)					
Pecan	1/8 pie	23.0	3.5	100	2
Pumpkin	1/8 pie	16.8	5.7	109	
Raisin	1/8 pie	12.9	3.1	0	1
Rhubarb	1/8 pie	17.1	4.5	2	3
Strawberry	1/8 pie	9.1	4.5	2	1
Sweet Potato	1/8 pie	18.2	6.0	70	2
Pie Tart, Fruit Filled	1	18.7	6.2	23	2
Popsicle	1 bar	0.0	0.0	0	0
Pudding					
Any Flavor Except Choc.	½ cup	4.3	2.5	70	0
Bread w/Raisins	½ cup	7.4	2.9	79	1
Choc. w/Whole Milk	½ cup	5.7	3.1	17	1
From Mix w/Skim Milk	½ cup	0.0	0.0	0	0
Rice w/Whole Milk	½ cup	4.4	2.5	16	1
Sugar Free Varieties	½ cup	2.2	1.4	10	0
Tapioca, w/2% Milk	½ cup	2.4	1.5	8	0
Pudding Pop, Frzn	1 bar	2.0	1.0	2	0
Sherbert	½ cup	1.0	0.5	7	0
Souffle, Choc.	½ cup	3.9	1.4	42	0
Strudel, Fruit	½ cup	1.2	0.1	2	1
Toppings					
Butterscotch/Caramel	3 T	0.1	0.0	0	0
Cherry	3 T	0.1	0.0	0	0
Choc. Fudge	2 T	4.0	2.0	0	0
Choc. Syrup, Hershey	2 T	0.4	0.2	0	0
Marshmallow	3 T	0.0	0.0	0	0
Milk Choc. Fudge	2 T	5.0	2.9	5	0
Pecans In Syrup	3 T	2.8	1.1	0	2
Pineapple	3 T	0.2	0.0	0	0
Strawberry	3 T	0.1	0.0	0	0
Whipped Topping					
Aerosol	¼ cup	3.6	1.4	0	0
From Mix	¼ cup	2.0	1.2	4	0
Frzn, Tub	¼ cup	4.8	3.6	0	0
Non-Fat	1 T	0.0	0.0	0	0

Desserts (continued)

Item	Serving	Tot. Fat (g)	Sat. Fat (g)	Chol. (mg)	Fiber (g)
Whipping Cream					
Heavy, Fluid	1 T	5.6	3.5	21	0
Light, Fluid	1 T	4.6	2.9	17	0
Turnover, Fruit Filled	1	19.3	5.4	2	1
Yogurt, Frozen					
Low-fat	½ cup	1.9	1.2	10	0
Nonfat	½ cup	0.0	0.0	0	0

Candy

Item	Serving	Tot. Fat (g)	Sat. Fat (g)	Chol. (mg)	Fiber (g)
Butterscotch					
Candy	6 pieces	1.3	0.4	0	0
Chips	1 oz.	8.3	6.8	0	0
Candied Fruit					
Apricot	1 oz.	0.1	0.0	0	1
Cherry	1 oz.	0.1	0.0	0	1
Citrus Peel	1 oz.	0.1	0.0	0	1
Figs	1 oz.	0.1	0.0	0	2
Candy Bar (Average)	1 oz.	8.5	4.5	5	1
Caramels					
Plain Or Choc. w/Nuts	1 oz.	4.6	2.2	10	0
Plain Or Choc. w/o Nuts	1 oz.	3.0	1.3	9	0
Choc.-Covered Cherries	1 oz.	4.9	2.9	1	1
Choc.-Covered Cream Center	1 oz.	4.9	2.6	1	1
Choc.-Covered Mint Patty	1 small	1.5	0.8	8	0
Choc.-Covered Peanuts	1 oz.	11.7	4.6	8	2
Choc.-Covered Raisins	1 oz.	4.9	2.9	3	1
Choc. Kisses	6 pieces	9.0	5.0	6	1
Choc. Stars	6 pieces	8.1	4.7	5	12
Cracker Jack	1 cup	3.3	0.4	0	0
English Toffee	1 oz.	2.8	1.7	5	
Fudge					
Choc.	1 oz.	3.4	1.5	1	0
Choc. w/Nuts	1 oz.	4.9	1.2	1	0

Item	Serving	Tot. Fat (g)	Sat. Fat (g)	Chol. (mg)	Fiber (g)
Gumdrops	28 pieces	0.2	0.0	0	0
Gummy Bears	1 oz.	0.1	0.0	0	0
Hard Candy	6 pieces	0.3	0.0	0	0
Jelly Beans	1 oz.	0.0	0.0	0	0
Licorice	1 oz.	0.1	0.0	0	0
Life Savers	5 pieces	0.1	0.0	0	0
M&M's					
Choc. Only	1 oz.	5.6	2.4	3	1
Peanut	1 oz.	7.8	2.4	4	1
Malted-Milk Balls	1 oz.	7.1	4.2	3	1
Marshmallow	1 large	0.0	0.0	0	0
Mints	14 pieces	0.6	0.0	0	0
Peanut Brittle	1 oz.	7.7	1.2	0	1
Peanut Butter Cups	1 oz.	9.2	3.6	3	1
Peppermint Pattie	1 oz.	3.0	2.0	0	<1
Raisinettes	1 oz.	5.5	3.0	4	0
Reese's Pieces	1.7 oz. pkg.	13.0	5.2	2	0
Sour Balls	1 oz.	0.0	0.0	0	0
Taffy	1 oz.	1.5	0.4	0	0
Tootsie Roll Pop	1 oz.	0.6	0.2	0	0
Tootsie Roll	1 oz.	2.3	0.6	0	1

FATS

Item	Serving	Tot. Fat (g)	Sat. Fat (g)	Chol. (mg)	Fiber (g)
Bacon Fat	1 T	14.0	6.4	0	0
Beef, Separable Fat	1 oz.	23.3	6.0	0	0
Butter					
Solid	1 t	3.8	2.4	0	0
Whipped	1 t	2.6	1.6	0	0
Butter Buds, Liquid	2 T	0.0	0.0	0	0
Butter Sprinkles	½ t	0.0	0.0	0	0
Chicken Fat, Raw	1 T	12.8	3.8	0	0
Cream					
Light	1 T	2.9	1.8	0	0
Medium (25% Fat)	1 T	3.8	2.3	0	0
Whipping, Light	1 T	4.6	2.9	0	0

FATS (CONTINUED)

Item	Serving	Tot. Fat (g)	Sat. Fat (g)	Chol. (mg)	Fiber (g)
Cream, Substitute					
Liquid/Frzn	½ fl. oz.	1.5	1.4	0	0
Powdered	1 T	0.7	0.7	0	0
Half & Half	1 T	1.7	1.1	0	0
Margarine					
Liquid Or Soft Tub	1 t	3.8	0.6	0	0
Reduced Calorie Tub	1 t	2.0	0.3	0	0
Solid (Corn), Stick	1 t	3.8	0.6	0	0
Fat-Free Tub	1 t	0.0	0.0	0	0
Mayonnaise					
Fat-Free	1 T	0.0	0.0	0	0
Reduced Calorie	1 T	5.0	0.7	0	0
Regular	1 T	12.0	1.3	0	0
No-Stick Spray (Pam, etc.)	2-sec spray	0.9	0.2	0	0
Oil					
Canola	1 T	13.6	1.0	0	0
Corn	1 T	13.6	1.7	0	0
Olive	1 T	13.5	1.8	0	0
Safflower	1 T	13.6	1.2	0	0
Soybean	1 T	13.6	2.0	0	0
Pork Fat (Lard)	1 T	12.8	5.0	0	0
Sandwich Spread (Miracle Whip Type)	1 T	4.9	0.7	0	0
Shortening, Vegetable	1 T	12.8	3.2	0	0
Sour Cream					
Cultured	1 T	3.0	1.9	0	0
Fat-Free	1 T	0.0	0.0	0	0
Half & Half, Cultured	1 T	1.8	1.1	0	0
Low-fat	1 T	1.8	1.1	0	0

FISH (ALL BAKED/BROILED W/O ADDED FAT UNLESS OTHERWISE NOTED)

Item	Serving	Tot. Fat (g)	Sat. Fat (g)	Chol. (mg)	Fiber (g)
Abalone, Canned	3 oz.	5.2	0.3	80	0
Anchovy, Canned In Oil	3 fillets	1.2	0.3	10	0
Bass					
Freshwater	3 oz.	4.5	0.9	60	0
Saltwater, Black	3 oz.	1.0	0.2	50	0
Saltwater, Striped	3 oz.	2.3	0.6	70	0
Bluefish					
Cooked	3 oz.	5.2	1.3	50	0
Fried	3 oz.	12.6	2.7	59	0
Butterfish					
Gulf	3 oz.	2.6	0.7	60	0
Northern	3 oz.	10.0	1.9	49	0
Carp	3 oz.	6.0	1.4	72	0
Catfish	3 oz.	3.0	0.7	60	0
Catfish, Breaded & Fried	3 oz.	13.0	2.9	75	1
Caviar, Sturgeon, Granular	1 t	1.5	0.4	47	0
Clams					
Canned, Solids & Liquid	½ cup	0.7	0.1	25	0
Meat Only	5 large	1.0	0.2	42	0
Soft, Raw	4 large	0.8	0.1	29	0
Cod					
Canned	3 oz.	0.6	0.2	45	0
Cooked	3 oz.	0.6	0.2	40	0
Dried, Salted	3 oz.	2.0	0.5	129	0
Crab					
Canned	½ cup	0.9	0.1	60	0
Deviled	3 oz.	10.0	3.5	40	0
Fried, Cake	3 oz.	18.0	4.1	170	0
Crab, Alaska King	3 oz.	1.2	0.2	53	0
Crab Cake	3 oz.	10.6	1.2	100	0
Crayfish, Freshwater	3 oz.	1.2	0.2	115	0
Croaker					
Atlantic	3 oz.	3.0	1.0	60	0
White	3 oz.	0.6	0.3	60	0
Dolphin Fish	3 oz.	0.8	0.2	72	0

Fish (continued)

Item	Serving	Tot. Fat (g)	Sat. Fat (g)	Chol. (mg)	Fiber (g)
Fillets, Frzn					
Batter Dipped	2 pieces	20.0	4.0	40	1
Breaded	2 pieces	18.0	3.0	35	1
Fish Cakes, Frzn, Fried	3 oz.	13.8	3.9	102	2
Flounder/Sole	3 oz.	0.4	0.2	30	0
Gefilte Fish	3 oz.	2.0	0.5	50	1
Grouper	3 oz.	1.2	0.3	45	0
Haddock					
Cooked	3 oz.	0.5	0.1	50	0
Fried	3 oz.	14.0	3.7	60	0
Halibut	3 oz.	1.0	0.5	30	0
Herring					
Canned Or Smoked	3 oz.	16.0	6.0	66	0
Cooked	3 oz.	11.0	2.0	70	0
Kingfish	3 oz.	3.0	0.8	68	0
Lobster					
Broiled With Butter	12 oz.	15.1	8.6	100	0
Steamed	3 oz.	0.5	0.1	70	0
Mackerel					
Atlantic	3 oz.	13.0	1.5	60	0
Pacific	3 oz.	12.5	1.7	55	0
Mussels, Meat Only	3 oz.	2.0	0.7	30	0
Ocean Perch					
Cooked	3 oz.	1.4	0.3	40	0
Fried	3 oz.	11.4	2.8	62	0
Octopus	3 oz.	2.0	0.4	95	0
Oysters					
Canned	3 oz.	2.0	0.8	54	0
Fried	3 oz.	13.7	3.2	83	0
Raw	5 – 8 med	1.8	0.6	54	0
Perch, Freshwater, Yellow	3 oz.	0.8	0.4	80	0
Pike					
Blue	3 oz.	0.7	0.5	75	0
Northern	3 oz.	1.0	0.7	40	0
Walleye	3 oz.	1.0	1.0	80	0
Pompano	3 oz.	9.5	5.0	55	0

Item	Serving	Tot. Fat (g)	Sat. Fat (g)	Chol. (mg)	Fiber (g)
Rainbow Trout					
Baked/Broiled	3 oz.	5.6	1.6	70	0
Breaded, Fried	3 oz.	14.4	3.2	84	1
Red Snapper	3 oz.	1.7	0.5	35	0
Rockfish, Oven Steamed	3 oz.	2.3	0.8	40	0
Roughy, Orange	3 oz.	2.0	0.1	20	0
Salmon					
Atlantic	3 oz.	6.2	0.9	55	0
Broiled/Baked	3 oz.	7.3	2.0	50	0
Chinook, Canned	3 oz.	7.0	2.0	50	0
Pink, Canned	3 oz.	5.0	1.3	54	0
Smoked	3 oz.	9.2	1.0	35	0
Sardines					
Atlantic, In Soy Oil	4 sardines	7.0	0.8	67	0
Skinless & Boneless	3 oz.	6.0	1.5	30	0
Scallops					
Cooked	3 oz.	1.0	0.2	30	0
Frzn, Fried	3 oz.	10.3	2.3	55	0
Steamed	3 oz.	1.2	0.2	40	0
Sea Bass, White	3 oz.	1.3	0.6	40	0
Shrimp					
Canned, Dry Pack	3 oz.	1.4	0.5	155	0
Canned, Wet Pack	3 oz.	0.6	0.3	125	0
Fried	3 oz.	10.5	0.9	120	0
Raw Or Broiled	3 oz.	1.0	0.5	150	0
Sole, Fillet	3 oz.	0.3	0.2	30	0
Squid					
Broiled	3 oz.	1.5	0.5	250	0
Fried	3 oz.	6.4	1.6	275	0
Raw	3 oz.	1.2	0.4	250	0
Sushi Or Sashimi	3 oz.	4.8	1.3	38	0
Swordfish	3 oz.	4.0	1.1	43	0
Trout					
Brook	3 oz.	3.5	0.9	60	0
Rainbow	3 oz.	7.5	1.2	85	0
Tuna					
Albacore	3 oz.	7.3	0.2	70	0
Canned, White In Oil	3 oz.	8.0	1.6	31	0

Fish (continued)

Item	Serving	Tot. Fat (g)	Sat. Fat (g)	Chol. (mg)	Fiber (g)
Tuna (continued)					
Canned, White In Water	3 oz.	1.5	0.5	25	0
Yellowfin	3 oz.	3.0	0.5	57	0
White Perch	3 oz.	3.7	0.7	65	0
Whiting	3 oz.	3.0	0.4	70	0
Yellowtail	3 oz.	5.2	0.9	75	0

Fruit

Item	Serving	Tot. Fat (g)	Sat. Fat (g)	Chol. (mg)	Fiber (g)
Apple					
Dried	½ cup	0.1	0.0	0	5
Whole w/Peel	1 medium	0.4	0.1	0	4
Applesauce, Unsweetened	½ cup	0.1	0.0	0	2
Apricots					
Dried	5 halves	0.2	0.0	0	6
Fresh	3 medium	0.4	0.0	0	2
Avocado					
California	1 (6 oz.)	30.0	4.5	0	4
Florida	1 (11 oz.)	28.0	4.3	0	4
Blackberries					
Fresh	1 cup	0.6	0.0	0	7
Frzn, Unsweetened	1 cup	0.7	0.0	0	7
Blueberries					
Fresh	1 cup	0.6	0.0	0	5
Frzn, Unsweetened	1 cup	0.7	0.2	0	4
Boysenberries, Frzn Unsweetened	1 cup	0.4	0.0	0	6
Cantaloupe	1 cup	0.4	0.0	0	3
Cherries	½ cup	0.8	0.2	0	2
Cranberries, Fresh	1 cup	0.2	0.0	0	4
Cranberry Sauce	½ cup	0.2	0.0	0	1
Dates, Whole, Dried	½ cup	0.4	0.0	0	8
Figs					
Canned	3 figs	0.1	0.0	0	9
Dried, Uncooked	10 figs	1.1	0.4	0	10
Fresh	1 medium	0.2	0.0	0	2

Item	Serving	Tot. Fat (g)	Sat. Fat (g)	Chol. (mg)	Fiber (g)
Fruit Cocktail, Canned w/ Juice	1 cup	0.3	0.0	0	5
Fruit Roll-Up	1	0.0	0.0	0	0
Grapefruit	½ med.	0.1	0.0	0	1
Grapes, Seedless	½ cup	0.1	0.0	0	1
Guava, Fresh	1 medium	0.5	0.2	0	7
Honeydew Melon, Fresh	¼ small	0.1	0.0	0	1
Kiwi, Fresh	1 medium	0.3	0.0	0	2
Kumquat, Fresh	1 medium	0.0	0.0	0	1
Lemon, Fresh	1 medium	0.2	0.0	0	1
Lime, Fresh	1 medium	0.1	0.0	0	1
Mandarin Oranges, Canned w/Juice	½ cup	0.0	0.0	0	4
Mango, Fresh	1 medium	0.6	0.0	0	4
Melon Balls, Frzn	1 cup	0.4	0.0	0	2
Mixed Fruit					
Dried	½ cup	0.5	0.0	0	5
Frzn, Unsweetened	1 cup	0.5	0.2	0	2
Nectarine, Fresh	1 medium	0.6	0.0	0	2
Orange					
Naval, Fresh	1 medium	0.1	0.0	0	4
Valencia, Fresh	1 medium	0.4	0.0	0	4
Papaya, Fresh	1 medium	0.4	0.1	0	3
Peach					
Canned, Water Pack	1 cup	0.1	0.0	0	4
Canned In Heavy Syrup	1 cup	0.1	0.0	0	4
Canned In Light Syrup	1 cup	0.1	0.0	0	4
Fresh	1 medium	0.1	0.0	0	1
Frzn, Sweetened	1 cup	0.3	0.0	0	4
Pear					
Canned In Heavy Syrup	1 cup	0.3	0.0	0	6
Canned In Light Syrup	1 cup	0.1	0.0	0	6
Fresh	1 medium	0.7	0.0	0	5
Persimmon, Fresh	1 medium	0.1	0.0	0	3
Pineapple Pieces					
Canned, Unsweetened	1 cup	0.2	0.0	0	2
Fresh	1 cup	0.7	0.0	0	3
Plantain, Cooked, Sliced	1 cup	0.2	0.0	0	2

Fruit (continued)

Item	Serving	Tot. Fat (g)	Sat. Fat (g)	Chol. (mg)	Fiber (g)
Plum					
Canned In Heavy Syrup	½ cup	0.1	0.0	0	4
Fresh	1 medium	0.4	0.0	0	3
Pomegranate, Fresh	1 medium	0.5	0.0	0	2
Prunes, Dried, Cooked	½ cup	0.2	0.0	0	10
Raisins					
Dark Seedless	½ cup	0.4	0.2	0	6
Golden Seedless	½ cup	0.4	0.2	0	6
Raspberries					
Fresh	1 cup	0.7	0.1	0	5
Frzn, Sweetened	1 cup	0.4	0.0	0	10
Rhubarb, Stewed, Unswetnd	1 cup	0.2	0.0	0	6
Strawberries					
Fresh	1 cup	0.6	0.0	0	3
Frzn, Sweetened	1 cup	0.3	0.0	0	3
Frzn, Unsweetened	1 cup	0.2	0.0	0	3
Tangerine, Fresh	1 medium	0.2	0.0	0	3
Watermelon, Fresh	1 cup	0.5	0.0	0	1

Fruit Juices

Item	Serving	Tot. Fat (g)	Sat. Fat (g)	Chol. (mg)	Fiber (g)
Apple Juice	1 cup	0.3	0.0	0	1
Apricot Nectar	1 cup	0.2	0.0	0	2
Carrot Juice	1 cup	0.4	0.0	0	2
Cranberry Juice Cocktail	1 cup	0.2	0.0	0	2
Cranberry-Apple Juice	1 cup	0.2	0.0	0	1.5
Grape Juice	1 cup	0.2	0.0	0	1
Grapefruit Juice	1 cup	0.2	0.0	0	1.5
Lemon Juice	2 T	0.0	0.0	0	0
Lime Juice	2 T	0.0	0.0	0	0
Orange Juice	1 cup	0.4	0.0	0	1
Peach Juice Or Nectar	1 cup	0.1	0.0	0	1
Pear Juice Or Nectar	1 cup	0.0	0.0	0	1
Pineapple Juice	1 cup	0.2	0.0	0	1
Prune Juice	1 cup	0.1	0.0	0	3
Tomato Juice	1 cup	0.2	0.0	0	2
V8 Juice	1 cup	0.1	0.0	0	2

LUNCH/DINNER COMBOS

Item	Serving	Tot. Fat (g)	Sat. Fat (g)	Chol. (mg)	Fiber (g)
Baked Bean w/Pork	½ cup	1.8	0.8	8	4
Beans					
Refried, Canned	½ cup	1.4	0.5	5	7
Refried, w/Fat	½ cup	13.2	5.2	12	7
Refried, Non-Fat	½ cup	0.0	0.0	0	7
Beans & Franks, Canned	1 cup	16.0	6.0	15	7
Beef & Vegetable Stew	1 cup	10.5	4.9	64	2
Beef Goulash w/Noodles	1 cup	13.9	3.6	87	2
Beef Noodle Casserole	1 cup	19.2	6.5	81	2
Beef Pot Pie	8 oz.	25.0	6.4	40	2
Beef Vegetable Stew	1 cup	10.5	5.0	64	2
Burrito					
Bean w/Cheese	1 large	11.0	5.4	26	4
Bean w/o Cheese	1 large	6.8	3.4	3	4
Beef	1 large	19.0	10.1	70	2
Cabbage Roll w/Beef & Rice	1 medium	6.0	2.7	26	2
Cannelloni, Meat & Cheese	1 piece	29.7	135.0	185	1
Cheese Souffle	1 cup	14.1	5.3	207	0
Chicken A La King, Hmde	1 cup	34.3	12.7	186	1
Chicken A La King w/Rice, Frzn	1 cup	12.0	4.0	122	1
Chicken & Dumplings	1 cup	10.5	2.7	103	1
Chicken & Rice Casserole	1 cup	18.0	5.1	103	1
Chicken & Veg. Stir-Fry	1 cup	6.9	1.2	26	3
Chicken Cacciatore, Frzn	12 oz.	11.0	3.8	80	1
Chicken Fricassee, Hmde	1 cup	18.1	5.2	85	1
Chicken-Fried Steak	4 oz.	23.4	6.8	115	0
Chicken Noodle Casserole	1 cup	10.7	3.2	59	2
Chicken Parmigiana, Hmde	7 oz.	17.0	5.9	150	2
Chicken Pot Pie	8 oz.	25.0	8.4	45	2
Chicken Salad, Regular	½ cup	21.2	9.1	56	0
Chicken Tetrazzini	1 cup	19.6	6.9	50	1
Chicken w/Cashews, Chinese	1 cup	28.6	4.9	60	2
Chili					
w/Beans Only	1 cup	12.0	4.0	35	7
w/Beans & Meat	1 cup	22.4	9.6	110	4

Lunch/Dinner Combos (continued)

Item	Serving	Tot. Fat (g)	Sat. Fat (g)	Chol. (mg)	Fiber (g)
Chop Suey w/Rice Or Noodles	1 cup	10.5	3.6	50	2
Chow Mein, Chicken	1 cup	6.0	2.5	60	2
Corned-Beef Hash	1 cup	24.4	7.5	80	2
Crab Cake	1 small	4.5	0.9	90	0
Creamed Chipped Beef	1 cup	23.0	7.9	44	0
Deviled Crab	½ cup	15.4	4.1	50	1
Deviled Egg	1 large	5.3	1.2	109	0
Egg Foo Yung w/Sauce	1 piece	7.0	1.9	107	1
Eggplant Parmesan, Traditional	1 cup	24.0	8.7	31	3
Egg Roll	2	6.8	2.4	40	1
Enchilada					
Bean, Beef & Cheese	8 oz.	14.1	7.3	38	3
Beef, Frzn	8 oz.	16.0	8.7	40	2
Cheese, Frzn	8 oz.	26.3	14.7	61	3
Chicken, Frzn	8 oz.	16.1	6.4	65	4
Fajitas					
Chicken	1	15.3	3.0	41	4
Beef	1	18.2	6.1	34	3
Fettuccine Alfredo	1 cup	29.7	9.3	73	3
Fish And Chips, Frzn Dinner	6 oz.	14.8	4.3	25	3
Fish Creole	1 cup	5.4	0.9	60	2
Frozen Dinner					
Beef Tips And Noodles	12 oz.	15.1	6.2	75	4
Chopped Sirloin	12 oz.	30.1	14.3	130	5
Fried Chicken	12 oz.	29.6	7.4	110	6
Meat Loaf	12 oz.	23.1	6.4	65	4
Salisbury Steak	12 oz.	27.4	13.5	126	4
Turkey And Dressing	12 oz.	22.6	5.0	74	3
Green Pepper Stuffed w/ Rice & Beef	1 medium	13.5	5.8	52	2
Hamburger Rice Casserole	1 cup	21.0	7.7	57	3
Ham Salad w/Mayo	½ cup	20.2	4.4	54	0
Lasagna					
Cheese	8 oz.	12.0	4.8	22	3
w/Beef & Cheese	1 piece	19.8	10.0	81	2

Item	Serving	Tot. Fat (g)	Sat. Fat (g)	Chol. (mg)	Fiber (g)
Lobster					
Cantonese	1 cup	19.6	5.6	240	0
Newburg	½ cup	24.8	14.7	183	0
Salad	½ cup	7.0	1.5	36	0
Lo Mein, Chinese	1 cup	7.2	1.4	11	1
Macaroni & Cheese	1 cup	16.0	5.0	20	0
Manicotti, Cheese & Tomato	1 piece	11.8	6.0	61	2
Meatball (Reg. Ground Beef)	1 med	5.1	2.0	30	0
Meat Loaf w/Reg. Ground Beef	3 oz.	20.2	8.5	102	0
Moo Goo Gai Pan	1 cup	17.2	3.1	66	1
Moussaka	1 cup	8.9	2.8	98	3
Onion Rings	10 average	17.0	6.0	0	1
Oysters Rockefeller	6 oysters	12.5	4.0	70	1
Pepper Steak	1 cup	11.0	3.2	53	1
Pizza					
Cheese	1 slice	10.1	5.2	40	1
Cheese, French Bread, Frzn	5 oz.	13.0	6.7	37	1
Combination w/Meat	1 slice	17.5	9.0	56	1
Deep Dish, Cheese	1 slice	13.5	6.9	45	1
Pepperoni	1 slice	16.5	8.5	44	1
Tomato Only	1 slice	4.0	2.0	2	1
Pizza Rolls, Frzn	3 pieces	6.9	2.0	10	1
Pork, Sweet & Sour w/Rice	1 cup	7.5	2.0	31	1
Quiche					
Lorraine	1/8 pie	43.5	20.1	218	1
Plain Or Vegetable	1 slice	17.6	8.8	135	1
Ratatouille	½ cup	3.0	0.7	0	2
Ravioli, Canned	1 cup	7.3	3.6	20	3
Ravioli w/Meat & Tomato Sauce	1 piece	3.0	0.9	19	0
Sailsbury Steak w/Gravy	8 oz.	27.3	12.3	126	1
Salmon Patty, Traditional	4 oz.	12.5	4.1	94	1

Lunch/Dinner Combos (continued)

Item	Serving	Tot. Fat (g)	Sat. Fat (g)	Chol. (mg)	Fiber (g)
Sandwiches (on whole wheat bread unless otherwise noted)					
BBQ Beef On Bun	1	16.8	5.8	54	4
BBQ Pork On Bun	1	12.2	3.7	56	4
BLT w/Mayo	1	15.6	4.1	23	4
Bologna & Cheese	1	22.5	9.7	42	4
Chicken w/Mayo And Lettuce	1	14.2	1.8	1191	4
Club w/Mayo	1	20.8	5.4	52	4
Corned Beef On Rye	1	10.8	3.2	34	4
Cream Cheese And Jelly	1	16.0	10.8	38	4
Egg Salad	1	12.5	2.5	228	4
French Dip, Au Jus	1	12.5	4.8	58	4
Grilled Cheese	1	24.0	12.4	56	4
Ham, Cheese & Mayo	1	16.0	7.3	29	4
Ham Salad w/Mayo	1	16.9	4.2	40	4
Peanut Butter & Jelly	1	15.1	2.3	10	5
Reuben	1	33.3	11.8	77	4
Roast Beef & Gravy	1	24.5	5.6	55	4
Roast Beef & Mayo	1	22.6	4.9	60	4
Sloppy Joe On Bun	1	16.8	5.8	54	4
Sub w/Salami & Cheese	1	41.3	17.7	109	4
Tuna Salad	1	17.5	2.9	17	4
Turkey & Mayo	1	18.4	1.9	17	4
Turkey Breast & Mustard	1	5.2	1.2	15	4
Shrimp Creole w/Rice	1 cup	6.1	1.2	123	2
Shrimp Salad	½ cup	9.5	1.6	69	1
Spaghetti					
w/Marinara Sauce	1 cup	2.5	1.0	5	2
w/Meat Sauce	1 cup	16.7	5.0	56	2
w/Red Clam Sauce	1 cup	7.3	1.0	17	2
w/Tomato Sauce	1 cup	1.5	0.4	5	2
w/White Clam Sauce	1 cup	19.5	2.6	49	1
Spaghettios	1 cup	2.0	0.5	8	2
Spinach Souffle	1 cup	14.8	7.1	184	2
Stroganoff					
Beef w/Noodles	1 cup	19.6	7.7	72	2
Beef w/o Noodles	1 cup	26.8	10.6	85	1

Item	Serving	Tot. Fat (g)	Sat. Fat (g)	Chol. (mg)	Fiber (g)
Sushi w/Fish & Vegetables	5 oz.	1.0	0.2	10	1
Taco, Beef	1 med	17.0	8.5	54	2
Tortellini, Meat Or Cheese	1 cup	15.4	5.4	238	1
Tostada w/Refried Beans	1 med	16.3	6.7	20	6
Tuna Noodle Casserole	1 cup	13.3	3.1	38	2
Tuna Salad					
Oil Pack w/Mayo	½ cup	16.3	2.7	20	0
Water Pack w/Mayo	½ cup	10.5	1.6	14	0
Veal Parmigiana	1 cup	22.5	10.1	75	0
Veal Scallopini	1 cup	20.4	7.3	132	2
Welsh Rarebit	1 cup	31.6	17.3	NA	0

MEATS (ALL COOKED W/O ADDED FAT UNLESS OTHERWISE NOTED)

Item	Serving	Tot. Fat (g)	Sat. Fat (g)	Chol. (mg)	Fiber (g)
Round, Eye Of, Lean	3 oz.	4.0	1.5	52	0
Beef, Lean, 5-10% Fat By Weight (Cooked)					
Flank Steak, Fat Trimmed	3 oz.	8.0	2.9	82	0
Hindshank, Lean	3 oz.	9.2	4.0	76	0
Porterhouse Steak, Lean	3 oz.	10.2	5.3	90	0
Rib Steak, Lean	3 oz.	9.2	5.0	80	0
Round Bottom, Lean	3 oz.	9.2	3.4	96	0
Roasted	3 oz.	7.2	2.7	81	0
Rump, Lean, Pot-Roasted	3 oz.	7.0	2.5	60	0
Top, Lean	3 oz.	6.2	2.2	89	0
Sirloin Steak, Lean	3 oz.	8.7	3.6	76	0
Sirloin Tip, Lean Roasted	3 oz.	9.2	3.9	90	0
Tenderloin, Lean, Broiled	3 oz.	11.0	4.2	83	0
Top Sirloin, Lean, Broiled	3 oz.	7.7	3.1	89	0
Beef, Regular 11-17.4% Fat By Weight (Cooked)					
Chuck, Separable Lean	3 oz.	15.0	6.2	105	0
Club Steak, Lean	3 oz.	12.7	6.1	90	0
Cubed Steak	3 oz.	15.2	3.3	85	0
Hamburger					
Extra Lean	3 oz.	13.9	6.3	82	0
Lean	3 oz.	15.7	7.2	78	0
Rib Roast, Lean	3 oz.	15.0	5.5	85	0
Sirloin Tips, Roasted	3 oz.	15.0	3.2	85	0

MEATS (CONTINUED)

Item	Serving	Tot. Fat (g)	Sat. Fat (g)	Chol. (mg)	Fiber (g)
Beef, Regular 11-17.4% Fat By Weight (Cooked) continued					
T-Bone, Lean Only	4 oz.	10.2	4.2	80	0
Tenderloin, Marbled	3 oz.	15.0	7.0	86	0
Beef, High Fat, 17.4-27.4% Fat By Weight (Cooked)					
Chuck, Ground	3 oz.	23.7	9.6	100	0
Hamburger, Regular	3 oz.	19.6	8.2	87	0
Meatballs	1 oz.	5.5	2.0	30	0
Porterhouse Steak, Lean & Marbled	3 oz.	19.5	8.2	80	0
Rib Steak	3 oz.	14.5	6.0	81	0
Rump, Pot-Roasted	3 oz.	19.5	8.2	80	0
Short Ribs, Lean	3 oz.	19.5	8.2	80	0
Sirloin, Broiled	3 oz.	18.5	7.7	78	0
Sirloin, Ground	3 oz.	26.5	9.3	84	0
T-Bone, Broiled	3 oz.	26.5	10.5	90	0
Beef, Highest Fat, = 27.5& Fat By Weight (Cooked)					
Brisket, Lean & Marbled	3 oz.	30.0	12.0	85	0
Chuck, Stew Meat	3 oz.	30.0	12.0	85	0
Corned, Medium Fat	3 oz.	30.0	14.9	75	0
Ribeye Steak, Marbled	3 oz.	38.6	12.0	90	0
Rib Roast	3 oz.	30.0	18.2	85	0
Short Ribs	3 oz.	31.5	10.5	90	0
Lamb					
Lean	3 oz.	8.0	3.4	100	0
Lean & Marbled	3 oz.	14.3	9.0	97	0
Loin Chop					
Lean	3 oz.	8.0	4.2	80	0
Lean & Marbled	3 oz.	22.3	11.7	58	0
Rib Chop					
Lean	3 oz.	8.0	5.0	50	0
Lean & Marbled	3 oz.	21.0	13.0	70	0
Liver					
Beef, Braised	3 oz.	4.8	1.9	400	0
Calf, Braised	3 oz.	6.8	2.3	450	0
Pork					
Bacon					
Cured, Broiled	1 strip	3.1	1.1	5	0

Item	Serving	Tot. Fat (g)	Sat. Fat (g)	Chol. (mg)	Fiber (g)
Pork (continued)					
Bacon (continued)					
Cured, Raw	1 oz.	16.3	6.0	19	0
Canadian Bacon, Broiled	1 oz.	1.8	0.6	14	0
Ham					
Cured, Canned	3 oz.	5.0	1.5	38	0
Cured, Shank, Lean	3 oz.	6.2	3.0	59	0
Marbled	2 slices	13.8	5.0	60	0
Fresh, Lean	3 oz.	6.3	1.5	40	0
Smoked	3 oz.	7.0	2.7	51	0
Smoked, 95% Lean	3 oz.	5.3	1.8	53	0
Loin Chop					
Lean	1 chop	7.7	3.0	55	0
Lean With Fat	1 chop	22.5	8.8	90	0
Rib Chop, Trimmed	3 oz.	9.8	3.5	81	0
Rib Roast, Trimmed	3 oz.	10.0	3.6	83	0
Sausage					
Brown And Serve	1 oz.	9.4	3.1	24	0
Patty	1	8.4	2.9	22	0
Regular Link	1/2 oz.	4.7	1.6	15	0
Sirloin, Lean, Roasted	3 oz.	10.0	3.6	85	0
Spareribs Roasted	6 med	35.0	11.8	121	0
Tenderloin, Lean, Roast	3 oz.	4.6	1.6	78	0
Top Loin Roast, Trimmed	3 oz.	7.5	2.8	77	0
Processed Meats					
Bacon Substitute (Breakfast Strips)	2 strips	4.8	1.0	0	0
Beef, Chipped	2 slices	1.1	0.4	15	0
Beef Breakfast Strips	2 strips	7.0	2.8	26	0
Beef Jerky	1 oz.	3.6	1.7	30	0
Bologna, Beef/Beef & Pork	2 oz.	16.2	6.9	33	0
Bratwurst					
Pork	2 oz link	22.0	7.9	51	0
Port & Beef	2 oz link	19.5	7.0	44	0
Chicken Roll	2 oz.	2.6	1.6	20	0
Corn Dog	1	20.0	8.4	37	0
Corned Beef, Jellied	1 oz.	2.9	1.0	3	0
Ham, Chopped	1 oz.	2.3	0.8	17	0

Meats (continued)

Item	Serving	Tot. Fat (g)	Sat. Fat (g)	Chol. (mg)	Fiber (g)
Hot Dog/Frank					
Beef	1	13.2	8.8	27	0
Beef, Fat-Free	1	0.0	0.0	0	0
Chicken	1	8.8	2.5	45	0
97% Fat-Free Varieties	1	1.6	0.6	22	0
Turkey	1	8.1	2.7	39	0
Turkey, Fat-Free	1	0.0	0.0	0	0
Knockwurst/Knackwurst	2 oz link	18.9	3.2	36	0
Pepperoni	1 oz.	13.0	5.4	25	0
Salami					
Cooked	1 oz.	10.0	6.6	30	0
Dry/Hard	1 oz.	10.0	3.0	16	0
Sausage					
Italian	2 oz link	17.2	6.1	52	0
90% Fat-Free Varieties	2 oz.	4.6	1.6	40	0
Polish	2 oz link	16.2	5.8	40	0
Smoked	2 oz link	20.0	9.2	48	0
Vienna	1 sausage	4.0	1.5	8	0
Turkey Breast, Smoked	2 oz.	1.0	0.3	23	0
Turkey Ham	2 oz.	2.9	1.0	32	0
Turkey Loaf	2 oz.	1.0	0.3	23	0
Turkey Roll, Light Meat	2 oz.	4.1	1.2	24	0
Veal					
Blade					
Lean	3 oz.	8.6	3.5	100	0
Lean With Fat	3 oz.	16.5	7.0	100	0
Breast, Stewed	3 oz.	18.5	8.7	100	0
Chuck, Med. Fat, Braised	3 oz.	12.6	6.0	101	0
Cutlet Breaded	3½ oz.	15.0	NA	NA	0

NUTS AND SEEDS

Item	Serving	Tot. Fat (g)	Sat. Fat (g)	Chol. (mg)	Fiber (g)
Almonds	2 T	9.3	1.0	0	2.5
Brazil Nuts	2 T	11.5	2.3	0	2.5
Cashews, Roasted	2 T	7.8	1.3	0	2
Chestnuts, Fresh	2 T	0.8	0.0	0	4
Hazelnuts (Filberts)	2 T	10.6	1.0	0	2
Macadamia Nuts, Roasted	2 T	12.3	2.0	0	2.5
Mixed Nuts					
w/Peanuts	2 T	10.0	1.5	0	2
w/o Peanuts	2 T	10.1	2.0	0	2
Peanut Butter, Creamy	1 T	8.0	1.5	0	1
Peanut Butter, Chunky	1 T	8.5	2.5	0	2
Peanuts					
Chopped	2 T	8.9	1.0	0	2
Honey Roasted	2 T	8.9	1.5	0	2
In Shell	1 cup	17.0	2.2	0	4
Pecans	2 T	9.1	0.5	0	1
Pine Nuts (Pignolia)	2 T	9.1	1.5	0	2
Pistachios	2 T	7.7	0.8	0	2
Poppy Seeds	2 T	3.8	0.3	0	2
Pumpkin Seeds	2 T	7.9	3.0	0	2
Sesame Nut Mix	2 T	5.1	1.5	0	2
Sesame Seeds	2 T	8.8	1.2	0	2
Sunflower Seeds	2 T	8.9	1.0	0	2
Trail Mix w/Seeds, Nuts, Carob	2 T	5.1	0.9	0	3
Walnuts	2 T	7.7	0.3	0	2.5

Pasta, Noodles and Rice

Item	Serving	Tot. Fat (g)	Sat. Fat (g)	Chol. (mg)	Fiber (g)
Macaroni					
Semolina	1 cup	0.7	0.0	0	1
Whole Wheat	1 cup	2.0	0.4	0	3.5
Noodles					
Alfredo	1 cup	25.1	9.8	73	1
Angel Hair	1 cup	1.5	0.5	0	0
Cellophone, Fried	1 cup	4.2	0.6	0	0
Chow Mein	1 cup	8.0	1.6	0	0
Egg	1 cup	2.4	0.4	50	1
Fettucine, Spinach	1 cup	2.0	0.5	0	2
Manicotti	1 cup	1.0	0.2	0	1
Ramen, All Varieties	1 cup	8.0	5.0	0	1
Rice	1 cup	0.3	0.0	0	1
Romanoff	1 cup	18.0	11.9	95	3
Spaghetti, Whole Wheat	1 cup	1.5	0.5	0	3
Spaghetti, Enriched	1 cup	1.0	0.0	0	1
Rice					
Brown	½ cup	0.6	0.0	0	2
Fried	½ cup	7.2	0.7	0	2
Long Grain & Wild	½ cup	2.1	0.2	0	1
Pilaf	½ cup	7.0	0.6	0	1
Spanish Style	½ cup	2.1	1.0	0	0
White	½ cup	1.2	0.0	0	0

POULTRY

Item	Serving	Tot. Fat (g)	Sat. Fat (g)	Chol. (mg)	Fiber (g)
Chicken					
Breast					
w/Skin, Fried	½ breast	10.7	3.0	87	0
w/o Skin, Fried	½ breast	6.1	1.5	90	0
w/Skin, Roasted	½ breast	7.6	2.9	70	0
w/o Skin, Roasted	½ breast	3.1	1.0	80	0
Leg					
w/Skin, Fried	1 leg	8.7	4.4	99	0
w/Skin, Roasted	1 leg	4.8	4.2	85	0
w/o Skin, Roasted	1 leg	2.5	0.7	41	0
Thigh					
w/Skin, Fried	1 thigh	11.3	2.5	60	0
w/Skin, Roasted	1 thigh	9.6	2.7	58	0
w/o Skin, Roasted	1 thigh	4.5	2.4	45	0
Wing					
w/Skin, Fried	1 wing	9.1	1.9	26	0
w/Skin, Roasted	1 wing	6.6	1.9	29	0
Duck					
w/Skin, Roasted	3 oz.	28.7	9.7	84	0
w/o Skin, Roasted	3 oz.	11.0	4.2	89	0
Turkey Breast					
Barbecued	3 oz.	3.0	1.3	42	0
Honey Roasted	3 oz.	2.6	1.1	38	0
Oven Roasted	3 oz.	3.0	1.3	42	0
Smoked	3 oz.	3.3	1.4	49	0
Turkey Dark Meat					
w/Skin, Roasted	3 oz.	11.3	3.5	89	0
w/o Skin, Roasted	3 oz.	7.0	2.4	75	0
Ground	3 oz.	13.2	4.0	85	0
Ham	3 oz.	5.0	1.7	62	0
Turkey Light Meat					
w/Skin, Roasted	3 oz.	8.2	2.3	76	0
w/o Skin, Roasted	3 oz.	3.2	1.0	55	0
Roll, Light Meat	3 oz.	7.0	2.0	43	0
Sliced w/Gravy, Frzn	3 oz.	3.7	1.2	20	0

Salad Dressings

Item	Serving	Tot. Fat (g)	Sat. Fat (g)	Chol. (mg)	Fiber (g)
Blue Cheese					
Fat-Free	1 T	0.0	0.0	0	0
Low Cal	1 T	1.9	0.2	2	0
Regular	1 T	8.0	1.4	0	0
Buttermilk, From Mix	1 T	5.8	1.0	5	0
Caesar	1 T	7.0	0.9	13	0
French					
Fat-Free	1 T	0.0	0.0	0	0
Low Cal	1 T	0.9	0.1	1	0
Regular	1 T	6.4	0.8	0	0
Garlic, From Mix	1 T	9.2	1.4	0	0
Honey Mustard	1 T	6.6	1.0	0	0
Italian					
Creamy	1 T	5.5	1.6	0	0
Fat-Free	1 T	0.0	0.0	0	0
Low Cal	1 T	1.5	0.1	1	0
Item	Serving	Tot. Fat (g)	Sat. Fat (g)	Chol. (mg)	Fiber (g)
Oil & Vinegar	1 T	7.5	1.5	0	0
Ranch Style	1 T	6.0	0.8	4	0
Russian					
Low Cal	1 T	0.7	0.1	1	0
Regular	1 T	7.8	1.1	0	0
Thousand Island					
Fat-Free	1 T	0.0	0.0	0	0
Low Cal	1 T	1.6	0.2	2	0
Regular	1 T	5.6	0.9	0	0

SAUCES AND GRAVIES

Item	Serving	Tot. Fat (g)	Sat. Fat (g)	Chol. (mg)	Fiber (g)
Barbecue Sauce	1 T	0.3	0.0	0	0
Bearnaise Sauce, Mix	¼ cup	25.6	15.7	71	0
Beef Gravy, Canned	½ cup	2.8	1.3	4	0
Brown Gravy					
From Mix	½ cup	0.9	0.4	1	0
Hmde	¼ cup	14.0	6.5	5	0
Catsup, Tomato	1 T	0.1	0.0	0	0
Chicken Gravy					
Canned	½ cup	6.8	1.7	3	0
From Mix	½ cup	0.9	0.3	1	0
Giblet, Hmde	¼ cup	2.6	0.7	28	0
Chili Sauce	1 T	0.0	0.0	0	0
Cocktail Sauce	¼ cup	0.2	0.0	0	0
Guacamole Dip	1 oz.	4.0	0.7	0	0
Hollandaise Sauce	¼ cup	18.0	10.2	160	0
Home-Style Gravy, From Mix	¼ cup	0.5	0.2	0	0
Horseradish	¼ cup	0.1	0.0	0	0
Jalepeno Dip	1 oz.	1.1	0.4	60	0
Mushroom Gravy					
Canned	½ cup	3.2	0.5	0	1
From Mix	½ cup	0.4	0.2	0	1
Mustard					
Brown	1 T	1.8	0.3	0	1
Yellow	1 T	0.7	0.0	0	0
Onion Dip	2 T	6.0	3.7	13	0
Onion Gravy, From Mix	½ cup	0.4	0.2	0	0
Pesto Sauce	¼ cup	29.0	7.3	18	1
Picante Sauce	½ cup	0.8	0.1	0	2
Pork Gravy, From Mix	½ cup	1.0	0.4	1	0
Sour-Cream Sauce	¼ cup	7.6	4.0	28	0
Soy Sauce	1 T	0.0	0.0	0	0
Soy Sauce, Reduced Sodium	1 T	0.0	0.0	0	0
Spaghetti Sauce					
"Healthy"/"Lite" Varieties	½ cup	1.0	0.0	0	3
Hmde, w/Ground Beef	½ cup	8.3	2.3	23	2
Marinara	½ cup	4.7	0.7	0	3

Sauces and Gravies (continued)

Item	Serving	Tot. Fat (g)	Sat. Fat (g)	Chol. (mg)	Fiber (g)
Spaghetti Sauce (continued)					
Meat Flavor, Jar	½ cup	6.0	1.0	5	2
Mushroom, Jar	½ cup	2.0	0.3	0	2
Oil & Garlic	½ cup	4.5	1.5	5	0
Tomato	½ cup	2.2	0.5	0	0
Spinach Dip (sour-cream & mayo)	2 T	7.1	1.8	10	1
Steak Sauce					
A-1	1 T	0.0	0.0	0	0
Others	1 T	0.0	0.0	0	0
Tabasco Sauce	1 t	0.0	0.0	0	0
Tartar Sauce	1 T	8.2	1.5	0	0
Teriyaki Sauce	1 T	0.0	0.0	0	0
Turkey Gravy					
Canned	½ cup	2.4	0.7	3	0
From Mix	½ cup	0.9	0.3	1	0
Worcestershire Sauce	1 T	0.0	0.0	0	0

Soups

Item	Serving	Tot. Fat (g)	Sat. Fat (g)	Chol. (mg)	Fiber (g)
Asparagus					
Cream of, w/Milk	1 cup	8.2	2.1	10	1
Cream of, w/Water	1 cup	4.1	1.0	5	1
Bean					
w/Bacon	1 cup	5.9	6.0	3	4
w/Ham	1 cup	8.5	2.0	3	3
w/o Meat	1 cup	3.0	1.5	2	5
Beef, Canned					
Broth	1 cup	0.5	0.2	1	0
Chunky	1 cup	5.1	2.6	14	2
Beef Barley	1 cup	1.1	0.5	6	1
Beef Noodle Casserole	1 cup	3.1	1.2	5	1
Black Bean	1 cup	1.5	1.2	0	2
Broccoli, Creamy w/Water	1 cup	2.8	1.0	5	1
Canned Vegetable w/o Meat	1 cup	1.6	0.6	0	1

Item	Serving	Tot. Fat (g)	Sat. Fat (g)	Chol. (mg)	Fiber (g)
Chicken					
Chunky	1 cup	6.6	2.0	30	2
Cream of, w/Milk	1 cup	11.5	4.6	27	0
Cream of, w/Water	1 cup	7.4	2.1	10	0
Chicken & Dumplings	1 cup	5.5	1.3	34	0
Chicken & Stars	1 cup	1.8	0.7	5	1
Chicken & Wild Rice	1 cup	2.3	0.5	7	1
Chicken/Beef Noodle or Veg.	1 cup	3.1	1.2	5	1
Chicken Gumbo	1 cup	1.4	0.3	5	1
Chicken Mushroom	1 cup	9.2	2.4	10	1
Chunky Chicken Noodle	1 cup	5.2	1.1	18	2
Chicken Noodle w/Water	1 cup	2.5	0.7	7	0
Chunky Chicken Vegetable	1 cup	4.8	1.4	17	2
Chicken Veggie w/Water	1 cup	2.8	0.9	10	0
Chicken w/Noodles, Chunky	1 cup	5.0	1.4	19	2
Chunky Chicken w/ Rice	1 cup	3.2	1.0	20	2
Chicken Rice w/Water	1 cup	1.9	0.5	7	1
Clam Chowder					
Manhattan Chunky	1 cup	3.4	2.1	14	1
New England	1 cup	6.6	3.6	7	1
Consomme w/Gelatin	1 cup	0.0	0.0	0	0
Corn Chowder	1 cup	10.5	5.0	22	3.5
Crab	1 cup	1.5	0.4	10	0
Fish Chowder, w/Whole Milk	1 cup	13.5	5.3	37	1
Gazpacho	1 cup	1.5	0.5	0	3
Seafood Gumbo	1 cup	3.9	2.7	40	3
Lentil	1 cup	1.0	0.2	0	3
Lobster Bisque	1 cup	14.0	5.5	35	1
Minestrone					
Chunky	1 cup	2.8	1.5	5	2
w/Water	1 cup	2.5	0.8	3	1
Mushroom, Cream of					
Condensed	1 cup	23.1	10.1	30	1
w/Milk	1 cup	13.6	5.1	20	1
w/Water	1 cup	9.0	2.4	2	1
Mushroom Barley	1 cup	2.3	0.4	0	1
Mushroom w/Beef Stock	1 cup	4.0	1.6	7	1

Soups (continued)

Item	Serving	Tot. Fat (g)	Sat. Fat (g)	Chol. (mg)	Fiber (g)
Onion	1 cup	1.7	0.3	0	1
Onion, French w/Cheese	1 cup	7.5	2.5	15	0
Oyster Stew w/Water	1 cup	3.8	2.5	14	1
Oyster Stew w/Whole Milk	1 cup	17.7	2.5	14	0
Pea					
Split	1 cup	0.6	0.2	1	1
Split w/Ham	1 cup	4.4	1.8	8	1
Potato, Cream of w/Milk	1 cup	7.4	1.2	5	2
Tomato					
w/Milk	1 cup	6.0	2.9	17	1
w/Water	1 cup	1.9	0.4	0	0.5
Tomato Beef w/Noodle	1 cup	4.3	1.6	5	1
Tomato Rice	1 cup	2.7	0.5	2	1
Turkey Noodle	1 cup	2.0	0.6	5	1
Turkey Vegetable	1 cup	3.0	0.9	2	1
Vegetable, Chunky	1 cup	3.7	0.6	0	2
Vegetable w/Beef, Chunky	1 cup	3.0	1.3	8	2
Vegetable w/Beef Broth	1 cup	1.9	0.4	2	1
Vegetarian Vegetable	1 cup	1.2	0.3	0	1
Wonton	1 cup	1.0	<1.0	10	1

Vegetables

Item	Serving	Tot. Fat (g)	Sat. Fat (g)	Chol. (mg)	Fiber (g)
Alfalfa Sprouts, Raw	½ cup	0.1	0.0	0	0
Artichoke, Boiled	1 medium	0.2	0.0	0	3
Artichoke Hearts, Boiled	½ cup	0.1	0.0	0	3
Asparagus, Cooked	½ cup	0.3	0.1	0	2
Avocado	½ cup	25.0	4.0	0	3.5
Bamboo Shoots, Raw	½ cup	0.2	0.1	0	2
Beans					
All Types, Cooked w/o Fat	½ cup	0.4	0.2	0	9
Baked, Brown Sugar & Molasses	½ cup	1.5	0.2	0	4
Baked, Vegetarian	½ cup	0.6	0.3	0	5
Baked w/Pork & Tomato Sauce	½ cup	1.3	0.5	8	5

Item	Serving	Tot. Fat (g)	Sat. Fat (g)	Chol. (mg)	Fiber (g)
Beets, Pickled	½ cup	0.1	0.0	0	4
Broccoli					
Cooked	½ cup	0.3	0.0	0	7
Frzn, Chopped, Cooked	½ cup	0.1	0.0	0	2
Frzn In Butter Sauce	½ cup	1.5	1.0	<5	2
Raw	½ cup	0.2	0.0	0	1
Brussel Sprouts, Cooked	½ cup	0.4	0.0	0	2
Butter Beans, Canned	½ cup	0.4	0.0	0	4
Cabbage					
Chinese (Bok Choy)	1 cup	0.2	0.0	0	2
Green, Cooked	½ cup	0.1	0.0	0	2
Carrot					
Cooked	½ cup	0.1	0.0	0	2
Raw	1 large	0.1	0.0	0	2
Cauliflower					
Cooked	1 cup	0.2	0.0	0	3
Raw	1 cup	0.1	0.0	0	4
Celery					
Cooked	½ cup	0.1	0.0	0	1
Raw	1 stalk	0.1	0.0	0	1
Chinese-Style Vegetables, Frzn	½ cup	4.0	0.2	0	3
Chives, Raw, Chopped	1 T	0.0	0.0	0	0
Collard Green, Cooked	½ cup	0.1	0.0	0	2
Corn					
Corn On The Cob	1 medium	1.0	0.1	0	4
Cream Style, Canned	½ cup	0.5	0.1	0	4
Frzn, Cooked	½ cup	0.1	0.0	0	4
Cucumber					
w/Skin	½ medium	0.2	0.0	0	1
w/o Skin, Sliced	½ cup	0.1	0.0	0	0
Eggplant, Cooked	½ cup	0.1	0.0	0	2
Green Beans					
French Style, Cooked	½ cup	0.2	0.0	0	2
Snap, Cooked	½ cup	0.2	0.0	0	2
Italian-Style Vegetables, Frzn	½ cup	5.5	0.2	0	2
Kale, Cooked	½ cup	0.3	0.0	0	2

Vegetables (continued)

Item	Serving	Tot. Fat (g)	Sat. Fat (g)	Chol. (mg)	Fiber (g)
Kidney Beans, Red, Cooked	½ cup	0.5	0.0	0	8
Leeks, Chopped, Raw	½ cup	0.1	0.0	0	1
Lentils, Cooked	½ cup	0.4	0.0	0	8
Lettuce, Leaf	½ cup	0.2	0.0	0	1
Lima Beans, Cooked	½ cup	0.4	0.0	0	5
Mushrooms					
Canned	½ cup	0.2	0.0	0	1
Raw	½ cup	0.2	0.0	0	1
Mustard Greens, Cooked	½ cup	0.2	0.0	0	2
Okra, Cooked	½ cup	0.1	0.0	0	3
Olives					
Black	3 med	4.5	0.5	0	1
Greek	3 med	5.0	0.9	0	1
Green	3 med	2.5	0.2	0	1
Onions					
Canned, French Fried	1 oz.	15.0	6.9	0	0
Chopped, Raw	½ cup	0.1	0.0	0	1
Parsley, Chopped, Raw	¼ cup	0.1	0.0	0	0
Peas, Green, Cooked	½ cup	0.2	0.0	0	4
Pickles	1 medium	0.1	0.0	0	0
Pepper, Bell, Chopped, Raw	½ cup	0.1	0.0	0	2
Pimentos, Canned	1 oz.	0.0	0.0	0	0
Potato					
Baked w/Skin	1 medium	0.2	0.1	0	4
Boiled w/o Skin	½ cup	0.1	0.0	0	2
French Fries	½ cup	6.8	3.0	10	2
Hash Browns	½ cup	10.9	3.4	23	2
Mashed w/Milk	½ cup	5.0	1.5	5	1
Potato Pancakes	1 cake	12.6	3.4	93	1
Scalloped	½ cup	6.0	3.5	12	1
Pumpkin, Canned	½ cup	0.3	0.2	0	4
Radish, Raw	½ cup	0.2	0.0	0	1
Rhubarb, Raw	1 cup	0.2	0.0	0	2
Sauerkraut, Canned	½ cup	0.2	0.0	0	4
Scallions, Raw	½ cup	0.2	0.0	0	4
Soybeans, Mature, Cooked	½ cup	7.7	1.1	0	4

Item	Serving	Tot. Fat (g)	Sat. Fat (g)	Chol. (mg)	Fiber (g)
Spinach					
Cooked	½ cup	0.2	0.1	0	3
Creamed	½ cup	5.1	0.7	1	3
Raw	1 cup	0.2	0.0	0	3
Squash	½ cup	0.2	0.0	0	3
Succotash, Cooked	½ cup	0.8	0.1	0	3
Sweet Potato					
Baked	1 medium	0.2	0.0	0	6
Candied	½ cup	3.4	1.2	8	5
Tempeh (Soybean Product)	½ cup	6.4	0.9	0	1
Tofu (Soybean Curd), Raw	½ cup	5.4	0.8	0	1
Tomato					
Boiled	½ cup	0.5	0.0	0	1
Raw	1 medium	0.4	0.0	0	1
Stewed	½ cup	0.2	0.0	0	1
Turnip Greens, Cooked	½ cup	0.2	0.0	0	2
Wax Beans, Canned	½ cup	0.2	0.0	0	2
Yam, Boiled/Baked	½ cup	0.1	0.0	0	3
Zucchini, Cooked	½ cup	0.1	0.0	0	2

Various Snacks

Item	Serving	Tot. Fat (g)	Sat. Fat (g)	Chol. (mg)	Fiber (g)
Cheese Puffs	1 oz.	10.0	4.8	14	0
Cheese Straws	4 pieces	7.2	6.4	5	1
Chex Snack Mix, Traditional	1 oz.	4.0	0.5	0	1
Corn Chips					
Barbecue	1 oz.	9.0	0.2	0	1
Regular	1 oz.	10.0	1.0	0	1
Cracker Jack	1 oz.	2.2	0.3	0	2
Mix (Cereal & Pretzels)	1 cup	2.5	0.5	0	2
Mix (Raisins & Nuts)	1 cup	25.0	3.5	1.5	4
Peanuts In Shell	1 cup	17.0	2.2	0	4
Popcorn					
Air Popped	1 cup	0.3	0.0	0	1
Caramel	1 cup	4.5	1.2	2	1
Microwave "Lite"	1 cup	1.0	0.0	0	1
Microwave, Plain	1 cup	3.0	0.7	0	1
Microwave, w/Butter	1 cup	4.5	1.8	1	1
Pork Rinds	1 oz.	9.3	3.7	24	0
Potato Chips					
Regular	1 oz.	11.2	2.9	0	1
Baked, Lays	1 oz.	1.5	0.0	0	2
Barbecue Flavor	1 oz.	9.5	2.6	0	1
Light, Pringles	1 oz.	8.0	2.0	0	0
Regular, Pringles	1 oz.	12.0	2.0	0	0
Pretzels (Hard)	1 oz.	1.5	0.5	0	1
Superpretzel® (Soft)	1 med.	1.0	0.0	0	2
Rice Cakes	1	0.0	0.0	0	0
Tortilla Chips					
Doritos	1 oz.	6.6	1.1	0	1
No Oil, Baked	1 oz.	1.5	1.0	0	1
Tostitos	1 oz.	7.8	1.1	0	1

Subject Index

35 Grams Fat/35 Grams Fiber Optional Meal Plans 37

A
Active Older Adults 229
Add Lots of Fiber to Your Diet 75

B
Bad Carbs & The Glycemic Index 55
Beat Food Cravings 131
Belly Fat Melting Tips 100
Best Fast Foods 123
Beware Restaurant Dining 125
Be Fit, Firm & Strong 236
BMI 164
Body-Shaping Plan 18
Body's Metabolism 7
Boost Metabolism to Burn Calories 175
Boost Your Energy Level 142
Boost Your Fat-Burning Metabolism 95
Bread and Flour 268
Breads, cereals, rice, and pasta 42
Breakfast Options 37
Build Muscle Mass 241

C
Calories Don't Count—Yes They Do! 117
Candy 278
Cardio and Strength Training Combo 262
Cereals 269

D
Daily Walk Keeps Arthritis Away 205
Dairy products 44, 271
Dance Fit-Step 143
Desserts 274
Detective's Walking Tips 181
Diet Fit-Step Mystery Clues 14, 31
Diet Fit-Step Strength-Training 248
Diet-Step®: 35/35 Meal Plans 23
Diet-Step® 35/35 Plan 14
Diet-Step®: Breakfast Options 37
Diets Don't Really Work 165

Dinner Options 40
Don't Stroke Out! 200
Double Blast of Calorie Burning 244
Dr. Walk's Fast Food Tips 122

E
Eating and Exercise 172
Eating When Away From Home 115
Eggs and egg substitutes 44, 272
Elliptical Fitness Machines 146
Exercise 47
Exercise and Arteries 204
Exercise and Brain Power 201
Exercise Decreases Risk of Breast & Uterine Cancer 206
Exercise Fallacies 138
Exercise Increases Your Appetite: Right?—Wrong! 174

F
Fast Eaters Gain Weight Faster 175
Fat & Fiber Counter 265
Fat Formula 164
Fat Makes You Fat! 83
Fats and oils 47, 279
Feel & Look Younger 216
Fiber Block Fats and Burn Calories 57
Fiber Decreases All Causes of Mortality 73
Final Clue, The 263
Fish 281
Fit-Step®: 35 Minute Plan 17
Fit-Step Mystery Walking Clues 151
Fit-Step® Mystery Walking Tips 140
Fitness in Adolescents & Young Adults 208
Fit-Step® Walk 188
Fit-Step Walking Workout 253
Fit-Step Workout Clues 249
Fit-Step Workout Exercise Tips 256
Flatten Your Abs with Power Breathing 224
Food Journal 118
French Paradox 72
Fruit 43, 284
Fruit Juices 286

307

G

Good High-Fiber Carbs 54

H

Harmful Protein 130
Have You Ever Seen a Runner Smile? 191
Healthy Antioxidant Secret Foods 70
Healthy Protein 128
Healthy Protein Meals 128
How About A Walk Just For Fun! 190
How Fiber Helps You Lose Weight 51
How Not to Have Fun! 191
How to Eliminate Dietary Trans Fats 89
How to Firm your Figure 225
How Trans Fats Increase Your Weight 88
How Your Body Burns Calories at Rest 221
How Your Body Burns Calories (Fuel) 7
How Your Body Changes Food Into Energy 8
How Your Body Stores Fuel 10

I

"I Don't Really Eat That Much!" 167
I'm Giving Up! Exercise Is Boring 157
Importance of Strengh-Training 240
Increase Fitness by Walking Up Hills 157
Indoor Diet Fit-Step® Plan 143
Interpreting Food Labels 265

K

Keeping Your Heart Healthy Through Good Nutrition and Exercise 41

L

Live Longer with Diet Fit-Step Plan 230
Lose Those Unwanted Pounds 217
Lose Weight with the Fit Step® 136
Lunch/Dinner Combos 287
Lunch Options 38

M

Mall Walking 147
Meat and meat substitutes 45, 291
Mediterranean Diet 70
Melt Belly Fat 99
Metabolic Mystery 127
Metabolic Syndrome: Fit or Fat? 98
Milk and Yogurt 272
Modern Day Diet Charlatans 4
More Advanced Walking Workouts 254
Mr. Fat's Accomplice Cholesterol 80
Mr. Fat's Hide-Out 82
The Mystery of 10,000 Steps 179
Mystery Clues for Shoes 155
Mystery Colors of the Spectrum 58
Mystery Diet Clues 109
The Mystery Diets of Two Countries 70
Mystery Drink 149
Mystery Muscle Builder 243
Mystery of the Fit-Step Stretch 227
Mystery Relaxation Plan 221
The Mystery of the Scale 132
Mystery Walking Cure 229
Mystery Weight-Loss Facts 103
The Mystery of Women 209
Myth of Cellulite 235

N

No More Unhealthy Diets 11
"No Pain – No Gain"—Not True! 193
Nuts and Seeds 43, 295

O

Once You're Fit, It Takes Longer to Get Out of Shape 261
Only 21 Days to Reach Your Peak 137
Other Common Exercise Myths 139
Oxygen: The Mystery Element 215

P

Pasta, Noodles and Rice 296
Portion Control 120
Potassium: Not Just For Runners 150
Poultry 297
Power Breakfast Without the Fat 95
Power Walk Off Those Unwanted Pounds 222
Prostate Cancer Patients Do Better With Exercise 207
Protein Diet Clues 128

Q

Quick Weight Loss Formula 22
Quick Weight-Loss Walking 168
Quick Weight-Loss Walking Snack Plan 170

R

Recumbent Stationary Bikes 145

S

Salad Dressings 298
Saturated Fat 85
Sauces and Gravies 299
Say No-No to Yo-Yo Diets 91
Say Yes-Yes to Walking 94
Skipping Fit-Step 147
Snacks 113, 306
Soups 45, 300
Stationary Bike Fit-Step 144
Stationary Fit-Step 143
Stay Motivated 157
Strengthen Bones and Muscles 223
Strength-Training Burns Fat 238
Sweets and desserts 46, 113
Swimming 147

T

Take a Happy Walk 156
Three Easy Steps to Everlasting Youth 219
Time Required to Walk Off Snacks 170
Travel Fit with the Fit-Step® 148
Treadmills 145
Trim-Step: Beach Toning 226
Turn Off the Mystery Machine 198
Types of Fats 85

U

Unsaturated Fats 86

V

Vegetables 43, 302

W

Walk Don't Run 192
Walking and Colon Cancer 206
Walking Burns Body Fat Not Carbohydrates 178
Walking Speed Predicts Longevity 212
Walking Around Keeps Blood Sugar Down 196
Walking For Fitness and Fun 153
Walking With Weights 245
Walk Away From High Blood Pressure 199
Walk Away From Type A 197
Walk Off Weight & Depression 203
Want to Lose Weight Faster? 166
What's the Best Time To Do the Fit-Step Workout? 260
What to Think About Before Eating 109
Why Women Gain Weight Easily 119
Worst Fast Foods 122

Y

You're Never Too Old to Strength Train 240

About The Author

Fred A. Stutman, M.D., has done extensive research in the fields of exercise physiology, diet, and nutrition at the U.S. Naval Air Development Center and in his private medical practice. As a medical officer in the U.S. Air Force, Dr. Stutman established one of the first walking programs for cardiac rehabilitation patients. Following the publication of *The Doctor's Walking Book*, he became known as "Dr. Walk."

Dr. Stutman is the author of eleven books and numerous medical articles on diet, nutrition, and exercise, which have been featured in *Prevention, Shape, Reader's Digest, Self, Family Circle, Star, Let's Live, Working Woman, Woman's World Weekly, First Magazine for Women, Ladies Home Journal, Cosmopolitan, Ms. Fitness, The National Enquirer, New York Times* and *USA Today*. Dr. Stutman has also appeared on national radio and TV, including The Today Show and Good Morning America.

Dr. Stutman is currently practicing Family Medicine as part of the Temple University Health System in Philadelphia. He is a Fellow of the American Academy of Family Practice and a recipient of the American Medical Association's Physician's Recognition Award. Dr. Stutman is also a member of the American College of Sports Medicine.